Gone

WITH THE

Fat

A COOKBOOK

BY

AVIS AND WARD NUTRITION ASSOCIATES

Copies may be obtained from:

Avis and Ward Nutrition Associates, Inc.
200 Professional Drive
West Monroe, LA 71291
(318)323-7949

First Printing December, 1994 - 5,000
Second Printing May, 1995 - 5,000
Third Printing September, 1995 - 10,000
Fourth Printing April, 1996 - 10,000
Fifth Printing August, 1996 - 10,000
Sixth Printing January, 1997 - 10,000
Seventh Printing May, 1997 - 20,000

ISBN: 0-962683-6-1

MANUFACTURED IN THE USA BY

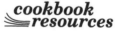

cookbook
resources

541 Doubletree Drive
Highland Village, Texas 75067
(972) 317-0205

COVER ARTIST:

James L. Kendrick, III is a Louisiana native, attended the University of Southwestern Louisiana, a former advertising manager, a Vietnam veteran and has been interested in art and painting since childhood. In 1974, with the encouragement of his wife, Edna, Mr. Kendrick turned his hobby as an artist into a full-time profession. Although his subject matter is not limited to any particular interest, Mr. Kendrick is best known for his antebellum plantation houses, scenes of old New Orleans and marine paintings. The painting on the cover is of Houmas House Plantation near Burnside, Louisiana and is available as a Limited Edition Print. For information/catalog on this and other prints by Mr. Kendrick contact:

Kendrick III Studio
34 Moselle Drive
Kenner, LA 70065
1-504-466-2084

ACKNOWLEDGMENTS

We want to thank all the people who have made this book possible and those who have shared their favorite recipes.

**Anne Hill Wood
Family and Friends
Coleen Cline - Divider Artist
Pen and Ink Magnolia**

TABLE OF CONTENTS

Introduction 6

Appetizers and Beverages 10

Dressings and Sauces 26

Soups and Salads 38

Entrees

    Fish and Seafood 70

    Poultry 92

    Beef 126

    Pork 147

    Game 152

    Vegetable 155

Vegetables and Starches 158

Breads 196

Desserts 220

The Good and The Bad 242

Nutritional Information

    Determining Goal Weight 264

    Determining Calorie Level 265

    Determining Fat Grams 265

    Estimating Fat Grams 266-271

    Menu Plans 272-273

    Trouble Shooter Guide 274

Nutrition Fact Sheet 275-276

    Foods to Order Out 280

    Substitution List 281

    Cooking Tips 282

    Getting Into Exercise 283

    The Importance of Water 284

    Equivalents 285-286

Index 287

Order Form 295

INTRODUCTION

Jen Avis and Kathy Ward believe there is not a better time to take charge of our health. For almost 14 years they have worked together in clinical nutrition. Both are registered licensed nutritionists in private practice.

Along with an established private practice, they have authored education materials, videos and cookbooks. Two previous books, *Southern But Lite* and *Just For Kids*, have enjoyed media coverage by *CNN*, ABC's *HomeShow*, *Good Morning America* and the *Gannet Wire*. The books have been widely distributed across the United States and abroad.

In 1992 Avis and Ward developed a low fat food line consisting of traditional Southern casseroles and desserts. They formulated their own fat-free soup base, making their products exclusively lower in fat than the typical prepared low fat cream soups found in the market.

The following example shows a comparison of Avis and Ward Soup Base to other popular low fat canned soups.

Avis and Ward Cream of Chicken - Less than 1 gram
Other Brands - 6 grams of fat

In a typical casserole as much as 2 cans of cream soups are used. Using Avis and Ward's soup bases lowers fat by as much as 10 grams per recipe. A product list is available at the back of the book if you desire to order or obtain information as to the availability of our food line. Leading companies are offering new products constantly. At Avis and Ward they believe low fat is not a trend, but here to stay!

To truly be successful, realistic but "tasty" changes must be made. If your family enjoys a particular Southern dish, this book will show you how converting it to low fat is not only easy, but your family will prefer it. See the Good and Bad Section for comparisons of "traditional" vs. "light" recipes. Also included are easy to follow methods to set up your own individualized program. Instructions for determining goal weight, caloric requirements and fat grams are in layman's terms. Whether your goal is weight loss, lowering cholesterol, decreasing heart disease risks, diabetes control or simply beginning to practice good nutrition, this book promises to offer fresh new choices. Avis and Ward Nutrition Associates, Inc. now presents:

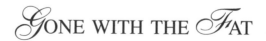

*G*ONE WITH THE *F*AT

Recipes were analyzed using the Nutritionist IV software. Hand calculations were used where adjustments were deemed necessary. All fat grams were rounded up to the nearest whole number.

EACH RECIPE LISTS: **Calories**
Cholesterol
Fat
Saturated Fat
Sodium
Dietary Fiber
Exchanges

SUBSTITUTIONS

IF HEALTHY CHOICE GROUND BEEF IS UNAVAILABLE IN YOUR AREA:

Use 80% lean ground beef and:
1. **Brown crumbled ground beef in skillet until no longer pink**
2. **Place crumbles in a colander**
3. **Rinse with hot water**
4. **Blot well with paper towels until dry**
5. **Proceed to use in recipe**

To prepare *"liquid butter substitute"*:
Mix 5½ tablespoons Butter Buds or Molly McButter to 1 cup water. Store in refrigerator in a sealed container.

APPETIZERS AND BEVERAGES

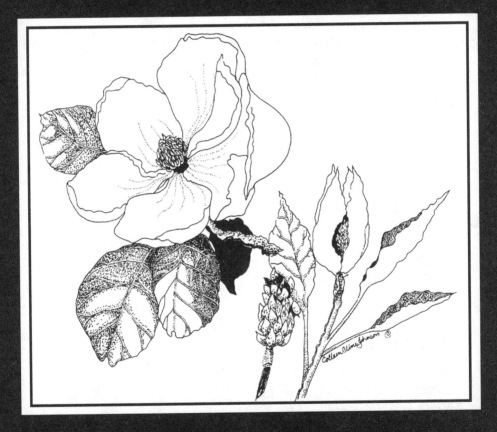

Colleen Cline Johnson ©

BROCCOLI CHEESE BARS

10 ounces chopped broccoli
1 tablespoon butter substitute granules
¾ cup egg substitutes
1 cup skim milk
¼ cup all purpose flour
¼ teaspoon salt
1 teaspoon baking powder
8 ounces light cheddar cheese
8 ounces fat free cheddar cheese
½ cup chopped onions
½ cup chopped mushrooms
   vegetable cooking spray

Spray a 13" x 9" pan with cooking spray. Thaw broccoli and squeeze out excess moisture. Mix all ingredients and spoon into pan. Bake in a preheated oven of 350 degrees F for 35 minutes or until lightly browned. Cool slightly. Cut into squares. Serve hot or at room temperature.

This may be served in larger portions as a side dish with a meal. Ten ounces frozen chopped spinach may also be substituted for the broccoli. This will not affect the nutritional specs.

Yield: 30 squares

Calories: 50
Exchanges: ½   *Meat*
                1   *Veg*

Cholesterol: 6   *Mg*
SF: <1 *Gm*
Fat: 1   *Gm*
Sodium: 221 *Mg*
Dietary Fiber: <1 *Gm*

CHEESE BALL

1 large package fat free cream cheese
1 large package light cream cheese
1 large can crushed pineapple
2 cups finely chopped green onions (do not use food processor)
4 ounces fat free cheddar cheese grated
¼ cup dried chives

Soften cream cheese at room temperature. Drain and press all juice out of crushed pineapple. Hand mix all ingredients in a bowl. Mix well. Form into a ball. Chill. Roll in chopped dried chives. Wrap in clear plastic. Keep refrigerated. Serve with fat free variety crackers.

Yield: 24 servings

Calories: 50
Exchanges: *½ Meat*

Cholesterol: *6   Mg*
SF: *1   Gm*
Fat: *2   Gm*
Sodium: *144 Mg*
Dietary Fiber: *0   Gm*

ARTICHOKE DIP

16 ounces frozen artichoke hearts
4 cloves garlic
½ cup fat free mayonnaise
12 ounces fat free cream cheese
1 cup Parmesan cheese grated
1 cup bread crumbs
½ package Italian salad dressing
1 tablespoon lemon juice
   vegetable cooking spray

Preheat oven to 375 degrees F. Combine finely chopped artichoke hearts and garlic. In a separate bowl, mix mayonnaise, cream cheese, lemon juice and ½ cup Parmesan cheese. Combine the two mixtures and pour into a 2 quart casserole that has been sprayed with vegetable cooking spray. Top with the remaining ½ cup of Parmesan cheese and bread crumbs. Bake for 20 minutes or until lightly browned and bubbly. Excellent served with fresh vegetables and toasted pita chips.

Yield: 16 servings

Calories: 79
Exchanges: *½* *Meat*
         1 *Veg*

Cholesterol: *9* *Mg*
SF: *1* *Gm*
Fat: *2* *Gm*
Sodium: *478 Mg*
Dietary Fiber: *2* *Gm*

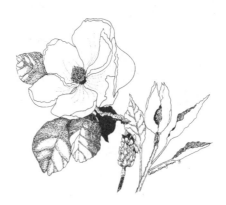

SPINACH AND CHEESE DIP

 1   envelope dry vegetable soup mix
16   ounces fat free sour cream
½   cup fat free mayonnaise
10   ounces frozen spinach
 4   ounces water chestnuts canned

Blend soup mix, sour cream and mayonnaise. Thaw and squeeze all excess moisture from spinach. Add to sour cream and mayonnaise mixture. Add chopped water chestnuts and stir to mix. Allow to chill for at least 2 hours. Serve with low fat or fat free crackers. This dip is very colorful served in a hollowed out purple cabbage or round loaf of brown bread.

Yield: 50 (tablespoon servings) or 5 cups total

Calories: 6
Exchanges: Free

Cholesterol: *0 Mg*
SF: *0 Gm*
Fat: *0 Gm*
Sodium: *26 Mg*
Dietary Fiber: 0 Gm

LIGHT CRAB DIP

2   cans crab meat
4   ounces light cheddar cheese
2   cups fat free mayonnaise
6   tablespoons fat free French salad dressing
2   teaspoons horseradish

Drain cans of crab. Rinse the crab meat. Mix all ingredients. Chill. Serve with fat free or low fat crackers.

Yield: 18 (4 Tablespoon) servings

Calories: 64
Exchanges: *½ Meat*
             ½ Bread

Cholesterol: *24 Mg*
SF: *<1 Gm*
Fat: *1 Gm*
Sodium: *580 Mg*
Dietary Fiber: 0 Gm

PICANTE DIP

8 ounces light cream cheese
1 can (16 ounces) picante sauce

Combine ingredients in a processor, blender or with an electric mixer. Served with baked tortilla chips. These can be found at the grocery store already prepared.

Yield: 48 tablespoons or 3 cups

Calories: 15
Exchanges: Free per 2 tablespoon serving

Cholesterol: 2   *Mg*
SF: 0   *Gm*
Fat: 1   *Gm*
Sodium: 155 *Mg*
Dietary Fiber: 0   *Gm*

TEX MEX DIP

16 ounces picante sauce or 2 (8 ounce) jars
16 ounces fat free sour cream
cilantro for garnish

Drain excess liquid from picante sauce, reserving 2 tablespoons of the liquid. Mix drained picante sauce and fat free sour cream. Stir in the two tablespoons of reserved liquid. Cover and chill. Garnish with fresh cilantro. Serve with fat free tortilla chips.

Yield • 16 (4 tablespoon) servings

Calories: 24
Exchanges: ½ *Meat*

Cholesterol: 0   *Mg*
SF: 0   *Gm*
Fat: 0   *Gm*
Sodium: 233 *Mg*
Dietary Fiber: 0   *Gm*

BRANDIED MEATBALLS

2   pounds Healthy Choice ground beef
¾   cup skim milk
2   slices light bread
1   tablespoon Worcestershire sauce
¼   teaspoon salt
½   teaspoon garlic powder
¼   teaspoon ground ginger
    dash of black pepper
½   teaspoon Tabasco
1   jar (18 ounces) apricot preserves
¼   cup brown sugar, packed
4   ounces brandy
1   tablespoon cornstarch
1   tablespoon water
    vegetable cooking spray

Combine the first 9 ingredients. Mix well. Shape into 1" meatballs. Cook meatballs in large skillet sprayed with cooking spray until browned. Combine preserves, brown sugar and brandy in a large skillet. Let simmer 10 minutes. Add meatballs. Cover and simmer for 1 hour. Stir occasionally. Combine cornstarch and water. Mix well. Stir into sauce. Stir constantly until sauce thickens slightly and bubbles.

Yield: 43 servings

Calories: 186
Exchanges: 2   *Meat*
               1   *Bread*
               1   *Veg*

Cholesterol: 6   *Mg*
SF: <1 *Gm*
Fat: <1 *Gm*
Sodium: 24 *Mg*
Dietary Fiber: <1 *Gm*

COCKTAIL MEATBALLS

1 pound Healthy Choice ground beef
2 tablespoons seasoned bread crumbs
¼ cup egg substitute
½ cup chopped bell pepper
½ cup chopped onions
vegetable cooking spray
1 can (10 ounces) tomatoes with hot chilies
¼ teaspoon sugar
2 tablespoons brown sugar, packed
3½ tablespoons Worcestershire sauce
1 tablespoons yellow mustard

Mix the Healthy Choice ground beef, bread crumbs and egg substitute. Shape into 50 meatballs. Place in an oblong baking dish that has been sprayed with cooking spray. Brown quickly in a 400 degree F oven. While meatballs are cooking, spray saucepan with cooking spray. Sauté bell peppers and onions until just tender, but still crisp. Add tomatoes, sugars, Worcestershire sauce and mustard. Mix well. Heat and pour over meatballs. Return to oven and bake at 300 degrees F for 20 minutes.

Yield: 50 meatballs (1 serving 2 meatballs)

Calories: 33
Exchanges: ½ *Meat*

Cholesterol: 9 *Mg*
SF: <1 *Gm*
Fat: 1 *Gm*
Sodium: 106 *Mg*
Dietary Fiber: <1 *Gm*

MEAT PIES

    vegetable cooking spray
8 ounces ground turkey sausage
8 ounces Healthy Choice ground beef
4 cans Pillsbury light biscuits
2 tablespoons chopped onions
    dash of pepper

Spray skillet with vegetable cooking spray. Add hamburger and sausage. Brown with onions and black pepper. Set aside. Open can of biscuits. Roll each biscuit into a flat circle. Place 1 tablespoon of meat mixture into the center of each flat biscuit. Fold dough over and seal the edges by pressing with a fork. Bake for 8 minutes at 425 degrees F.

Yield: 40 servings

Calories: 69
Exchanges: *½ Meat*
                ½ Bread

Cholesterol: *8 Mg*
SF: *<1 Gm*
Fat: *2 Gm*
Sodium: *228 Mg*
Dietary Fiber: *1 Gm*

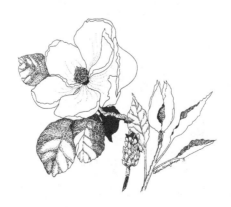

STUFFED MUSHROOMS

24   mushroom caps
     vegetable cooking spray
1½   cups crab meat
1   ounce liquid Butter Buds
¼   lemon juice
     dash of red pepper
1   cup medium white sauce

Preheat oven to 350 degrees F. Cook onions and crab meat in butter substitute liquid until warm. Stir in white sauce (see index for medium white sauce recipe.) Spray mushroom caps with butter flavored cooking spray and fill. Bake in shallow baking dish prepared with cooking spray for 10 - 15 minutes.

Yield: 24 mushrooms

Calories: 13
Exchanges: *½*   *Meat for 3 mushrooms*

Cholesterol: *9*   *Mg*
SF: *0*   *Gm*
Fat: *0*   *Gm*
Sodium: *76*   *Mg*
Dietary Fiber: *0*   *Gm*

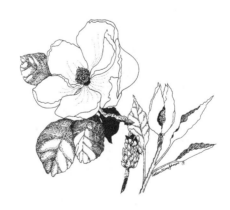

PIZZA SNACK

1 fat free tortilla
3 tablespoons fat free spaghetti sauce
2 teaspoons onions chopped
¼ cup fat free Mozzarella cheese grated
2 teaspoons fat free Parmesan cheese
olive oil flavored cooking spray
2 teaspoons bell pepper chopped

Spray tortilla with olive oil flavored cooking spray. Bake sprayed tortilla on a baking sheet at 400 degrees F for 3 minutes. Remove from oven. Leaving ½" around the edge, spread spaghetti sauce, onion, bell pepper, oregano and cheeses. Bake 5 minutes at 400 degrees F until cheese is brown.

Yield: 1 serving

Calories: 164
Exchanges: *1   Meat*
               1   Bread
               ½   Veg

Cholesterol: *8   Mg*
SF: *0   Gm*
Fat: *0   Gm*
Sodium: *420 Mg*
Dietary Fiber: *2   Gm*

SHRIMP COCKTAIL FOR A CROWD

½ **pound shrimp raw**
8 **ounces fat free cream cheese**
4 **ounces tomato catsup**
1 **tablespoon prepared horseradish**
1 **tablespoon Worcestershire sauce**

Boil shrimp in Rex liquid shrimp boil. Peel and devein. (Or you may choose to substitute 8 ounces of frozen shrimp or a small can of shrimp. This will affect the sodium) While shrimp cool in the refrigerator, lay cream cheese on an attractive plate. Allow cheese to come to room temperature. Blend the catsup, horseradish and Worcestershire sauce. Pour over cream cheese. Just before serving, place shrimp on top of cream cheese and sauce. Surround with low fat or fat free crackers.

Yield: 12 servings

Calories: 49
Exchanges: ½   *Meat*

Cholesterol: 32 *Mg*
SF: 0   *Gm*
Fat: <1 *Gm*
Sodium: 250 *Mg*
Dietary Fiber: 0   *Gm*

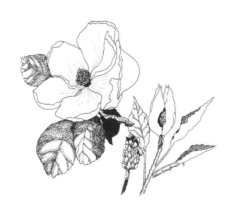

CAFÉ VIENNESE

1 cup instant decaffeinated coffee
1 cup sugar
⅔ cup dry non fat milk
½ teaspoon cinnamon

Combine ingredients, and mix well. Store in airtight container. For each serving, place 2 rounded teaspoons of mix into a cup. Add 1 cup of boiling water and stir. You may wish to serve with a cinnamon stick stirrer.

Diabetics may leave out sugar. Use 1 rounded teaspoon per cup and add 1 package of Sweet and Low or Equal, reducing the calories to 7. This will make a free food.

Yield: 48 servings

Calories: 23

Cholesterol:	*<1*	*Mg*
SF:	*0*	*Gm*
Fat:	*0*	*Gm*
Sodium:	*5*	*Mg*
Dietary Fiber:	*0*	*Gm*

ORANGE CAPPUCCINO

½ cup instant decaffeinated coffee
¾ cup sugar
½ teaspoon dehydrated orange peel
1 cup dry non fat milk

Combine first four ingredients and mix well. Store mix in an airtight container. For each serving use ½ tablespoon of mix to 1 cup boiling water. Stir until blended.

To make sugar free Orange Cappuccino, leave out sugar and put only 2 teaspoons of mix per cup. This will reduce the calories by 20, making a free food choice for diabetics.

Yield: 24 servings

Calories: 38
Calories with sugar: 76

Cholesterol:	*1*	*Mg*
SF:	*0*	*Gm*
Fat:	*0*	*Gm*
Sodium:	*16*	*Mg*
Dietary Fiber	*0*	*Gm*

SWISS MOCHA COFFEE

½ cup instant decaffeinated coffee
½ cup sugar
2 tablespoons dry cocoa
1 cup dry non fat milk

Combine first four ingredients and mix well. Store mix in an airtight container. For each serving use 1 tablespoon plus 1 teaspoon of mix to 1 cup boiling water. Stir until blended.

Diabetics may leave out the sugar. Put only 2 teaspoons of mix and one package of Equal or Sweet and Low in cup of boiling water. This will reduce calories by 20 and make a free food choice for diabetics.

Yield: 24 servings

Calories: 31
Cholesterol: *½ Mg*

SF: *0 Gm*
Sodium: *16 Mg*
Fat: *0 Gm*
Dietary Fiber: 0 Gm

OLD-FASHIONED STRAWBERRY SODA

10 ounces frozen strawberries
24 ounces diet creme soda
4 tablespoons light Cool Whip
3 cups fat free vanilla ice cream

Mash strawberries with a fork. Add 1 cup ice cream and ½ cup creme soda. Stir Well. Spoon equal amounts of this mixture into 4 tall (14 ounce) glasses. Top with remaining ice cream and fill glasses with remaining soda. Garnish each glass with a tablespoon of light Cool Whip. If available, garnish with a sprig of mint.

Yield: 4 servings

Calories: 176
Exchanges: *2 Bread*
                 1 Fruit

Cholesterol: *<1 Mg*
SF: *0 Gm*
Fat: *2 Gm*
Sodium: *140 Mg*
Dietary Fiber: 2 Gm

QUICK FRUIT PUNCH

1   can (46 ounces) pineapple juice
1   can (46 ounces) orange juice
1   can (46 ounces) apple juice
1   package unsweetened cherry powdered drink mix
1   cup sugar

Combine pineapple, orange and apple juices. Gradually add drink mix. Add 1 cup sugar. Chill for several hours.

Yield: 25 cups

Calories: 122
Exchanges: Not acceptable for diabetics.

Diabetics may substitute 24 packages of sugar substitute for sugar.
Calories: 95
Exchanges: 1 Fruit

Cholesterol: 0   Mg
SF: 0   Gm
Fat: 0   Gm
Sodium: 6   Mg
Dietary Fiber: 0   Gm

WHITE GRAPE PUNCH

12   ounces white grape juice concentrate
12   ounces frozen lemonade
96   ounces (3, 32 ounce bottles) club soda

Combine white grape juice and lemonade concentrate with club soda. Stir until dissolved. Chill.

Yield: 25 cups

Calories: 32
Exchanges: 1   Fruit

Cholesterol: 0   Mg
SF: 0   Gm
Fat: 0   Gm
Sodium: 6   Mg
Dietary Fiber: 0   Gm

DEEP SOUTH WASSAIL

8   cups apple cider
2   cups unsweetened orange juice
1   cup lemon juice
4   cups unsweetened pineapple juice
1   teaspoon whole cloves
4   tablespoons honey

Combine all ingredients and bring to a simmer. Strain and serve hot.

A wonderful Christmas beverage

Yield: 24 servings

Calories: 91
Exchanges: *1*   *Fruit*

Cholesterol: *0*   *Mg*
SF: *0*   *Gm*
Fat: *0*   *Gm*
Sodium: *4*   *Mg*
Dietary Fiber: *0*   *Gm*

MUSCADINE WINE

4   cups sugar
1   package yeast
1   can (12 ounces) grape juice concentrate or 32 ounces
   muscadine juice
1   can (6 ounces) lemonade concentrate
   water

Mix all ingredients well. Add enough water to fill a gallon jug 2 inches below the neck of the jug. Place a balloon on top of the jug and let stand for 21 days. Strain the wine through cheese cloth into bottles and cork.

Yield: 32 (4 ounce) servings

Calories: 128
Exchanges: Not acceptable for diabetics.

Cholesterol: *0*   *Mg*
SF: *0*   *Gm*
Fat: *0*   *Gm*
Sodium: *4*   *Mg*
Dietary Fiber: *<1*   *Gm*

DRESSINGS AND SAUCES

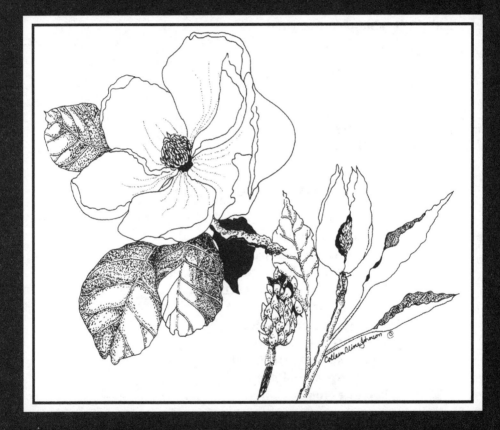

BAR-B-Q SAUCE

½ cup diet cola
¼ cup catsup
1 tablespoon liquid smoke
1 tablespoon mustard
¼ teaspoon onion powder
¼ teaspoon garlic powder

Mix all ingredients well.

Yield: 12 (1 tablespoon) servings

Calories: 7

Cholesterol:	*0*	*Mg*
SF:	*0*	*Gm*
Fat:	*0*	*Gm*
Sodium:	*73*	*Mg*
Dietary Fiber:	*<1*	*Gm*

SOUTHERN BAR-B-Q SAUCE

4½ tablespoons cider vinegar
¼ cup lemon juice
½ cup Worcestershire sauce
2 tablespoons brown sugar, packed
3 tablespoons yellow mustard
2¼ teaspoons salt
1½ teaspoons apple juice
3 cups tomato catsup
1 tablespoon garlic powder
1 tablespoon red pepper
12 ounces tomato puree

Blend all ingredients in a large saucepan. Heat until mixture almost boils.

Yield: 149 tablespoon servings or 2⅓ quarts

Calories: 8 per tablespoon

Cholesterol:	*0*	*Mg*
SF:	*0*	*Gm*
Fat:	*0*	*Gm*
Sodium:	*105*	*Mg*
Dietary Fiber:	*<1*	*Gm*

EASY SALSA

1   can (16 ounces) stewed tomatoes
1   can (15 ounces) Rotel tomatoes
¼   teaspoon garlic powder

Put tomatoes and garlic powder in blender. Pulse two to three times, just to blend. Let sit 30 minutes for flavors to blend

Yield: 32 (1 tablespoon) servings

Calories: 6
Exchanges: Free

Cholesterol: *0*   *Mg*
SF: *0*   *Gm*
Fat: *0*   *Gm*
Sodium: *89*   *Mg*
Dietary Fiber: *<1*   *Gm*

CHEESE SAUCE

2   cups thin white sauce
2   ounces light American cheese

Make thin white sauce. (See Thin White Sauce in index of this book). Cube cheese. When sauce comes to a boil, add cheese. When mixture becomes creamy, it is ready. Great over vegetables, baked potatoes, homemade pasta, macaroni and in casseroles.

Yield: 36 (1 tablespoon) servings

Calories: 14
Exchanges: Free

Cholesterol: *1*   *Mg*
SF: *<1*   *Gm*
Fat: *<1*   *Gm*
Sodium: *106 Mg*
Dietary Fiber: *<1*   *Gm*

CRANBERRY WINE SAUCE

1   can (16 ounces) cranberry sauce
¼   cup red table wine
2   tablespoons brown sugar, packed
1   tablespoon mustard
¼   teaspoon garlic powder

Combine all ingredients in a saucepan. Simmer uncovered for 5 minutes. Serve hot or cold with turkey, chicken or pork.

Yield: 2½ cups or 40 teaspoon servings

Calories: 27

Cholesterol:	*0*	*Mg*
SF:	*0*	*Gm*
Fat:	*0*	*Gm*
Sodium:	*10*	*Mg*
Dietary Fiber:	*0*	*Gm*

FAT FREE HOLLANDAISE SAUCE

¾   cup fat free mayonnaise
1   tablespoon lemon juice
½   cup evaporated skim milk
    dash of black pepper

Combine fat free mayonnaise, skim evaporated milk, lemon juice and pepper in a saucepan. Simmer. Simmer to blend until thickened.

Yield: 1¼ cups (10, 2 tablespoon servings)

Calories: 28
Exchanges: Free

Cholesterol:	*<1*	*Mg*
SF:	*0*	*Gm*
Fat:	*0*	*Gm*
Sodium:	*259*	*Mg*
Dietary Fiber:	*0*	*Gm*

SPINACH SALAD DRESSING

2   tablespoons olive oil
⅔   cup olive juice (liquid from jar of olives)
⅓   cup wine vinegar
1   cup minced onion
3   tablespoons prepared mustard
½   teaspoon garlic powder
½   teaspoon celery seeds

Pour all ingredients into blender on high for a few seconds. Keep refrigerated. Reblend before using. Best when used over a fresh spinach salad.

Yield: 2 cups (16, 2 tablespoon servings)

Calories: 27
Exchanges: Free

Cholesterol: *0   Mg*
SF: *<1 Gm*
Fat: *2   Gm*
Sodium: *58 Mg*
Dietary Fiber: 0   Gm

MAMA B'S THOUSAND ISLAND DRESSING

1   cup fat free mayonnaise
¼   cup tomato catsup
1   teaspoon yellow mustard
1   tablespoon sweet pickle relish
2   hard boiled egg whites
¼   teaspoon black pepper
1   tablespoon dehydrated onion flakes

Mix all ingredients.

Yield: 25 (1 tablespoon) servings

Calories: 13
Exchanges: Free

Cholesterol: *0   Mg*
SF: *0   Gm*
Fat: *<1   Gm*
Sodium: *165 Mg*
Dietary Fiber: <1   Gm

OLE SOUTH COATING MIX

4 cups white bread crumbs
1 tablespoon salt
1 tablespoon paprika
1 teaspoon garlic powder
1 tablespoon celery powder

Mix all ingredients well. Cover and seal. Place in refrigerator to store.

HINTS ON HOW TO USE A COATING MIX:

Blend in ½ cup egg substitute, ½ cup mix. Dip meat. Dredge through the coating mix. Bake meats at 375 degrees F until done. Lemon pepper, dried herbs, sesame and poppy seeds may be added depending on preference. Great for chicken, fish and lean meats. Spray food with vegetable cooking spray before placing on baking dish.

Yield: 34 (2 tablespoon) servings

Calories: 18
Exchanges: Free

Cholesterol: *0*   *Mg*
SF: *0*   *Gm*
Fat: *0*   *Gm*
Sodium: *231 Mg*
Dietary Fiber: *0*   *Gm*

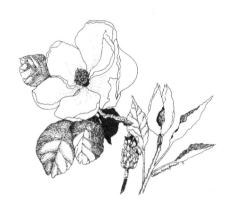

GRAVY FOR CHICKEN OR BEEF

1   can (16 ounces) defatted chicken or beef broth
2   tablespoons cornstarch

Put can of broth in refrigerator for an hour or two before using. Remove and open. Skim off any fat that has hardened on the top. This will eliminate much of the fat.

Blend broth and cornstarch. Bring to a boil. After mixture has boiled for 1 or 2 minutes, it is ready.

Yield: 16 (2 tablespoon) servings

Calories: 7
Exchanges: Free

Cholesterol: 0   Mg
SF: 0   Gm
Fat: 0   Gm
Sodium: 42   Mg
Dietary Fiber: 0   Gm

SWEET AND SOUR MARINADE

1   cup salt free soy sauce
½   cup unsweetened pineapple juice
½   cup vinegar
½   cup sugar
¼   teaspoon garlic powder

Combine all ingredients. Store in a Mason or canning jar. Will keep in refrigerator up to 6 months. Excellent for basting chicken, pork or turkey. Can be used in stir fry recipes for vegetables or meat and vegetables

Yield: 2½ cups (or 40 tablespoons)

Calories: 18
Exchanges: Free

Cholesterol: 4   Mg
SF: 0   Gm
Fat: 0   Gm
Sodium: 265 Mg
Dietary Fiber: 0   Gm

FAT FREE ROUX

1 cup all purpose white flour

OVEN METHOD:

Place 1 cup flour in cast iron skillet or Dutch oven. Bake at 400 degrees F until dark brown or the color of a copper penny. Stir about every 15 minutes. 3 - 4 cups of flour may be browned at one time, then stored in a quart canning jar or other container that seals well.

MICROWAVE METHOD:

Place 1 cup of flour in Pyrex casserole dish. Microwave on high for 2 minutes. Stir well. Repeat at 1 minute intervals until flour is dark brown, about the color of a copper penny. Small amounts do best in the microwave.

This fat free roux may be used to thicken and color gumbos, coat meats (roasts, center cut port chops or chicken) and in gravies.

Yield: 16 (1 tablespoon) servings

Calories: 28
Exchanges: ½ *Bread*

Cholesterol: 0 *Mg*
SF: 0 *Gm*
Fat: <1 *Gm*
Sodium: <1 *Mg*
Dietary Fiber: <1 *Gm*

SPORTSMAN'S SAUCE

1	can (16 ounces) tomato sauce
¼	cup Worcestershire sauce
¼	cup lemon juice
12	ounces catsup
2	teaspoons Kitchen Bouquet
1	tablespoon yellow mustard
1	tablespoon chili powder
1	cup onion chopped
1	teaspoon garlic powder
1	can light beer
½	cup liquid Butter Buds
	Tabasco sauce to taste

Mix all ingredients. Simmer on low heat 20 - 30 minutes.

Excellent on any wild game such as lean venison or as a basting sauce for grilling meat, poultry or fish.

Yield: 30 (2 tablespoon) servings

Calories: 26
Exchanges: Free

Cholesterol: *0*   *Mg*
SF: *0*   *Gm*
Fat: *<1*   *Gm*
Sodium: *288*   *Mg*
Dietary Fiber: *1*   *Gm*

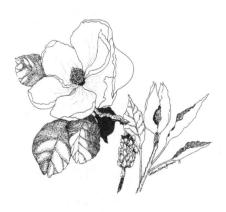

MEDIUM WHITE SAUCE

3   ounces liquid Butter Buds
¼   teaspoon salt
⅛   teaspoon white pepper
⅛   teaspoon black pepper
2   cups skim milk
2   tablespoons cornstarch

CONVENTIONAL METHOD:

Mix cornstarch and milk until smooth. Add liquid Butter Buds, salt and pepper. Stir constantly. Bring to a boil over medium heat. Boil for 1 minute.

MICROWAVE METHOD:

Put milk and cornstarch in a microwave safe bowl. Stir until smooth. Add liquid Butter Buds, salt and pepper. Microwave on high. Stir twice with fork or wire whisk for 3 - 5 minutes or until mixture boils. Boil 1 minute.

Cornstarch has twice the thickening power of flour and is lower in carbohydrates and calories. For these reasons it is a preferred substitute for flour.

Yield: 2 cups (32 tablespoon servings)

Calories: 8
Exchanges: Free per tablespoon for diabetics.

Cholesterol: *<1 Mg*
SF: *0   Gm*
Fat: *0   Gm*
Sodium: *58 Mg*
Dietary Fiber: *0   Gm*

THIN WHITE SAUCE

3 ounces liquid Butter Buds
¼ teaspoon salt
⅛ teaspoon white pepper
⅛ teaspoon black pepper
2 cups skim milk
1 tablespoon cornstarch

CONVENTIONAL METHOD:

Mix cornstarch and milk until smooth. Add liquid Butter Buds, salt and pepper. Stir constantly. Bring to a boil over medium heat. Boil for 1 minute.

MICROWAVE METHOD:

Put milk and cornstarch in a microwave safe bowl. Stir until smooth. Add liquid Butter Buds, salt and pepper. Microwave on high. Stir twice with fork or wire whisk for 3 - 5 minutes or until mixture boils. Boil 1 minute.

Cornstarch has twice the thickening power of flour and is lower in carbohydrates and calories. For these reasons it is a preferred substitute for flour.

Yield: 2 cups (32 tablespoon servings)

Calories: 8
Exchanges: Free per tablespoon for diabetics.

Cholesterol:	*<1*	*Mg*
SF:	*0*	*Gm*
Fat:	*0*	*Gm*
Sodium:	*58*	*Mg*
Dietary Fiber:	*0*	*Gm*

THICK WHITE SAUCE

6 **ounces liquid Butter Buds**
¼ **teaspoon salt**
⅛ **teaspoon white pepper**
⅛ **teaspoon black pepper**
2 **cups skim milk**
4 **tablespoons cornstarch**

CONVENTIONAL METHOD:

Mix cornstarch and milk until smooth. Add liquid Butter Buds, salt and pepper. Stir constantly. Bring to a boil over medium heat. Boil for 1 minute.

MICROWAVE METHOD:

Put milk and cornstarch in a microwave safe bowl. Stir until smooth. Add liquid Butter Buds, salt and pepper. Microwave on high. Stir twice with fork or wire whisk for 3 - 5 minutes or until mixture boils. Boil 1 minute.

Cornstarch has twice the thickening power of flour and is lower in carbohydrates and calories. For these reasons it is a preferred substitute for flour.

Yield: 2 cups (32 tablespoon servings)

Calories: 11
Exchanges: Free per tablespoon for diabetics.

Cholesterol: *<1 Mg*
SF: *0 Gm*
Fat: *0 Gm*
Sodium: *91 Mg*
Dietary Fiber: 0 Gm

SOUPS AND SALADS

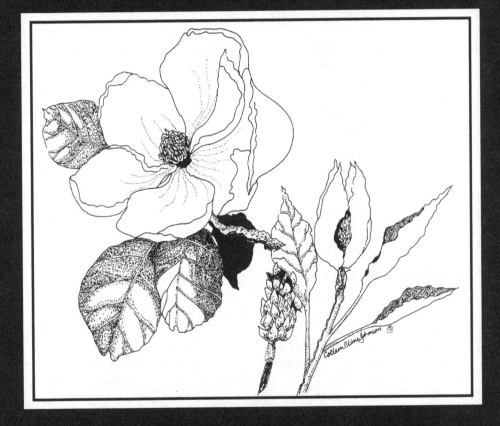

JACK'S BEAN SOUP

2 cups A & W soup mix (see index for page listing)
½ pound Healthy Choice turkey sausage
½ cup chopped onions
5 ounces Rotel tomatoes with chilies
2 cloves garlic
¼ teaspoon salt
8 cups water

A & W BEAN SOUP MIX:

1 pound packages each of the following dried beans/peas
   navy beans
   baby lima beans
   large lima beans
   great Northern beans
   red kidney beans
   black beans
   lentils
   barley
   split peas
   black eyed peas

Mix all beans. Store in a sealed container.

Yield: makes 10 (2 cup) servings

SOUP:

Cover 2 cups dry A & W bean soup mix with water. Let sit overnight or at least 2 hours. Drain. Chop onions and garlic. Set aside. Cut link sausage into ¼ inch slices. Place beans and all ingredients into a large saucepan or crockpot. Add water. Bring to a boil. Lower heat and simmer 2 hours.

12 (1 cup) servings

Calories: 71
Exchanges: *½ Meat*
                 1   Bread

Cholesterol: *9   Mg*
SF: *0   Gm*
Fat: *1   Gm*
Sodium: *294 Mg*
Dietary Fiber: 2   Gm

OYSTER BISQUE

- 16 ounces raw oysters
- 3 cups 2% low fat milk
- 1 cup evaporated skim milk
- ¼ cup chopped onions
- ½ cup celery chopped
- 1 teaspoon dried parsley
- 1 bay leaf
- 4 ounces liquid butter substitute
- ⅓ cup all purpose flour
- ¼ teaspoon salt
- ½ teaspoon Tabasco sauce

Drain oysters, reserving 1 cup liquid. Pour liquid into saucepan. Cut oysters into several small pieces. Add oysters to saucepan. Slowly bring oysters to just before the boiling point, (do not boil). Take off stove. In Pyrex dish, scald milks, onion, celery, parsley and bay leaf in microwave for 2 minutes on high. Add liquid butter substitute. Blend flour, salt and Tabasco sauce with a small amount of oyster liquid until smooth. Slowly stir back into larger quantity of oysters and liquid. Remove bay leaf. Heat to serving temperature. Garnish with chopped green onion.

Yield: 8 (1 cup) servings

Calories: 132
Exchanges: ½   *Meat*
               ½   *Bread*
               1   *Milk*

Cholesterol: 22 *Mg*
SF: 1 *Gm*
Fat: 3 *Gm*
Sodium: 436 *Mg*
Dietary Fiber: <1 *Gm*

VEGETABLE CHEDDAR CHOWDER

3   cups water
3   bouillon cubes
4   cubed potatoes
1   cup chopped onion
1   cup sliced carrots
½   cup chopped bell peppers
2   ounces dry butter substitute granules
⅓   cup flour
⅓   cup skim milk
10 ounces grated fat free cheddar cheese
2   ounces pimientos
¼   teaspoon Tabasco sauce

Combine water and bouillon cubes in a Dutch oven. Bring to a boil. Add vegetables. Cover and simmer 15 minutes or until vegetables are tender. Blend flour and milk in large canning jar. Secure lid. Shake until flour and milk are well mixed. Pour flour mixture into vegetable mixture. Simmer and cook over low heat until cheese melts.

Yield: 4 (1 cup) servings

Calories: 134
Exchanges: *1*   *Meat*
                 1   *Bread*
                 1   *Veg*

Cholesterol: *5*   *Mg*
SF: *<1*   *Gm*
Fat: *<1*   *Gm*
Sodium: *241*   *Mg*
Dietary Fiber: *2*   *Gm*

BOUILLABAISSE (FISH CHOWDER)

2½   pounds red snapper fillets
2   cups diced peeled tomatoes
1   cup diced celery
½   cup diced bell pepper
5   cloves garlic
     olive oil flavored cooking spray
1   tablespoon olive oil
½   teaspoon salt
½   teaspoon black pepper
1/5   teaspoon red pepper

Season fish and set aside. Spray heavy skillet with cooling spray and drizzle with oil. Arrange half of onion, celery and garlic in a layer. Arrange half of sliced tomatoes and fish in a layer. Then repeat layers. Place covered pot on low heat and simmer for 1½ hours. Do not stir. To keep from scorching, lift pot from stove occasionally, and holding it in both hands, rotate. This should be done every 10 - 15 minutes.

Yield: 10 servings

Calories: 143
Exchanges: *4   Meat*
                1   Veg
                ½   Fat

Cholesterol: *41 Mg*
SF: *1   Gm*
Fat: *3   Gm*
Sodium: *390 Mg*
Dietary Fiber: *1   Gm*

CAJUN GAZPACHO

30	ounces vegetable juice cocktail
1	cup cucumber diced
1	cup tomato diced
1	tablespoon sugar
¼	cup red table wine
1	tablespoon olive oil
10	green onions finely chopped
¼	teaspoon red pepper
1	clove garlic

Blend together in a food processor, 2 cups of vegetable juice cocktail, ½ cup cucumber, ½ cup tomato, sugar, red wine, olive oil, red pepper and garlic. Add the processed vegetables to the remainder of the vegetable cocktail and cucumbers and tomatoes. Add the green onions. Serve very cold.

Yield: 6 (¾ cup) servings

Calories: 78
Exchanges: *2* *Veg*

Cholesterol: *0* *Mg*
SF: *<1* *Gm*
Fat: *2* *Gm*
Sodium: *830* *Mg*
Dietary Fiber: *2* *Gm*

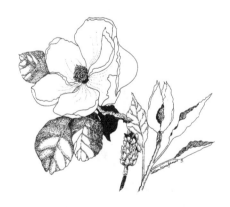

LOW FAT VICHYSSOISE

     vegetable cooking spray
 2   cups chopped onions
 3   cups cubed potatoes
 32 ounces fat free chicken broth
 13 ounces skim evaporated milk
 ¼   teaspoon black pepper

Spray large saucepan with cooking spray. Add onions. Cook until tender. Do not brown. Add potatoes and chicken broth to onions. Cook until potatoes are soft. Cool. Put in blender or food processor and blend. Add evaporated milk. Heat slowly. Add pepper to taste. This soup can be served hot or cold. Soup tastes better when made the day before.

Yield: 10 servings

Calories: 107
Exchanges: *1*   *Bread*
            ½   *Veg*

Cholesterol: *1*   *Mg*
SF: *<1*   *Gm*
Fat: *1*   *Gm*
Sodium: *182* *Mg*
Dietary Fiber: *2*   *Gm*

INSTANT POTATO SOUP

 4   cups water
 2   chicken bouillon cubes
 2   servings instant potato flakes
 1   tablespoon dried onion flakes
     dash of black pepper

Bring water, onion flakes and black pepper to a boil. Remove saucepan from burner. Add potato flakes while stirring.

Yield: 4 (1 cup) servings

Calories: 58
Exchanges: *1*   *Bread*

Cholesterol: *0*   *Mg*
SF: *<1*   *Gm*
Fat: *<1*   *Gm*
Sodium: *454* *Mg*
Dietary Fiber: *<1*   *Gm*

HEARTY POTATO SOUP

4 **ounces Healthy Choice honey ham, chopped**
¼ **cup liquid Butter Buds**
½ **cup diced celery**
1 **cup chopped onions**
6 **cups diced potatoes**
8 **cups skim milk**
vegetable cooking spray

Spray a saucepan with vegetable cooking spray. Add butter buds, onion, chopped ham and celery. Cook until onion and celery are soft. Set aside. Cook potatoes in pan covered with water until soft. Drain. Add all ingredients to one large pot and simmer. For thicker soup add 2 tablespoons cornstarch. Cook 1 hour.

Yield: 8 servings

Calories: 258
Exchanges: ½ *Meat*
2 *Bread*
1 *Milk*

Cholesterol: 10 *Mg*
SF: 1 *Gm*
Fat: 1 *Gm*
Sodium: 380 *Mg*
Dietary Fiber: 4 *Gm*

TURNIP SOUP

2 cups peeled and diced turnips
1 cup potatoes, diced
1 cup onion, chopped
½ cup liquid Butter Buds
1½ tablespoons all purpose flour
3 cups fat free chicken broth
1 cup evaporated skim milk
1 tablespoon chopped parsley

In a Dutch oven or a stock pot, cook turnips and potatoes in liquid Butter Buds until tender. Approximately 20 - 30 minutes. Sprinkle in flour and blend thoroughly. Pour in broth. Mix well. Bring to a boil. Reduce heat and simmer for 15 minutes. Cool soup and blend until smooth in blender. Reheat and add milk. Serve topped with fresh parsley.

Yield: 6 servings

Calories: 111
Exchanges: ½ *Bread*
2 *Veg*

Cholesterol: 2 *Mg*
SF: <1 *Gm*
Fat: 1 *Gm*
Sodium: 483 *Mg*
Dietary Fiber: 2 *Gm*

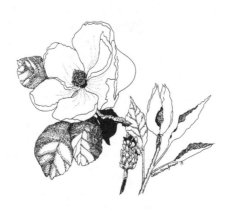

FRESH MUSHROOM SOUP

1	cup chopped onions
½	cup shredded carrot
3	cubes beef bouillon
6	cups water
3	tablespoons chopped parsley
1	clove garlic
½	teaspoon black pepper
1	cup diced celery
¾	pound sliced fresh mushrooms
8	ounces low fat Mozzarella cheese
4	tablespoons liquid Butter Buds
	butter flavored cooking spray

In a soup pot dissolve beef cubes in water. Bring to a boil. Add onion, carrot and celery and cook until vegetables are tender. Puree until tender. Return soup to pot. In a skillet, sauté mushrooms in butter flavored spray until tender. Add mushrooms and all remaining ingredients except the Mozzarella cheese. Cook 15 to 20 minutes. Ladle into soup bowls. Sprinkle 1 ounce cheese into each bowl.

Yield: 12 servings

Calories: 93
Exchanges: *1   Meat*
               ½   Veg

Cholesterol: *0   Mg*
SF: *2   Gm*
Fat: *3   Gm*
Sodium: *177 Mg*
Dietary Fiber: *1   Gm*

QUICK SEAFOOD GUMBO

2 cups chopped onion
1 chopped bell pepper
2 cups diced celery
2 cans fat free beef broth
2 cups sliced okra
16 ounce can stewed tomatoes
¼ teaspoon red pepper
½ pound crab meat
½ pound peeled, raw shrimp
2 cups water
   vegetable cooking spray
   dash of salt

Sauté onions, pepper and celery in non-stick vegetable spray until clear. Add defatted beef broth, water, tomatoes and okra. Simmer until done. Add crab meat and shrimp and season with red pepper and salt. Simmer 30 minutes. Serve over rice.

Yield: 8 servings

Calories: 111
Exchanges: *1½ Meat*
         2 Vegs

Cholesterol: *59 Mg*
SF: *<1 Gm*
Fat: *2 Gm*
Sodium: *373 Mg*
Dietary Fiber: *2 Gm*

FRENCH ONION SOUP

1	cup chopped onions
1	can defatted beef broth
1½	cups water
2	tablespoons Worcestershire sauce
¼	teaspoon black pepper
4	ounces light Swiss cheese
1	plain bagel
	butter flavored cooking spray

Spray saucepan with cooking spray. Add onion. Cook 5 to 6 minutes until lightly browned. Add broth, water and Worcestershire sauce. Simmer 10 to 15 minutes. While soup is simmering, chip up bagel (see instructions below) and place bagel chips into four bowls and top with one ounce of Swiss cheese. When soup is done, ladle over chips and cheese in bowl.

BAGEL CHIPS:

Slice bagels in food processor. Spray chips with butter flavored cooking spray and arrange on baking sheet. Bake at 200 degrees F for 25 minutes. Let cool. The chips should be crisp. You may be able to find prepared bagel chips in the stores, but be sure to check label for added fat.

Yield: 4 (1 cup servings)

Calories: 172
Exchanges:

1	*Meat*
½	*Bread*
½	*Veg*
½	*Fat*

Cholesterol:	*20*	*Mg*
SF:	*3*	*Gm*
Fat:	*5*	*Gm*
Sodium:	*780*	*Mg*
Dietary Fiber:	*1*	*Gm*

SPLIT PEA SOUP

16	ounces dried split peas
2	quarts water
1	cup onion, chopped
1	carrot, diced
1	potato, (1 ounce) diced
8	ounces Healthy Choice ham
¼	teaspoon salt
¼	teaspoon black pepper
¼	teaspoon ground tarragon

Wash and sort peas. Cover with water about 2 inches over the peas. Soak overnight. Drain peas. Add 2 quarts water, vegetables, ham and seasonings. Bring to a boil. Cover. Reduce heat and simmer for 3 hours. Stir occasionally. If soup becomes too thick, add water. This soup may be made in a crockpot.

Yield: 12 (1 cup) servings

Calories: 169
Exchanges: *1*   *Meat*
             1½ Bread

Cholesterol: *9*   *Mg*
SF: *<1 Gm*
Fat: *1*   *Gm*
Sodium: *60 Mg*
Dietary Fiber: *4*   *Gm*

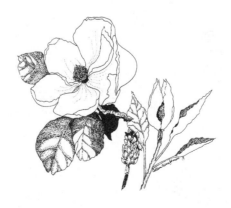

SHRIMP CORN SOUP

1 cup all purpose flour
1 cup chopped onions
1 rib chopped celery
1 cup chopped bell pepper
1 clove garlic
1 gallon water
1 can (16 ounces) whole canned tomatoes
8 ounces canned tomatoes
24 ounces frozen corn kernels
1 teaspoon salt
½ teaspoon black pepper
2 pounds peeled raw shrimp
1 tablespoon dried parsley
  vegetable cooking spray

Spray large saucepan with cooking spray. Heat and sauté onion, celery, bell pepper and garlic. Cook, stirring often until vegetables are tender. Mix cup of fat free roux with 2 cups of warm tap water. Gradually add hot tap water to vegetable mixture. (You may want to put roux and water into a jar with a tight lid and shake to mix and pour over vegetable mixture). Add tomatoes, tomato sauce, corn and seasonings. Bring to a boil. Reduce heat. Simmer about 1 hour. Add shrimp and parsley to soup. Bring back to a boil and cook an additional 10 minutes. Serve with cornbread or hot French bread.

Yield: 12 servings

Calories: 188
Exchanges:　2　*Meat*
　　　　　　　1　*Bread*
　　　　　　　1　*Veg*

Cholesterol:　117 *Mg*
SF:　　　　　1　*Gm*
Fat:　　　　　2　*Gm*
Sodium:　　　426 *Mg*
Dietary Fiber: 2　*Gm*

VEGETABLE SOUP

4 cups cubed raw potato
2 cups mixed frozen vegetables
1 can (16 ounces) stewed tomatoes
¼ teaspoon garlic powder
1 cup chopped onions
3 cans (30 ounces) fat free, reduced sodium chicken broth
vegetable cooking spray
1 cup diced celery

Spray large saucepan with cooking spray. Heat. Add onion, celery and cook until onion becomes transparent. Add remaining ingredients. Bring to a boil. Reduce heat and simmer for about an hour.

May substitute defatted beef broth with 1 pound Healthy Choice ground beef for a more hearty soup. Calories 240, Fat 3 gm, per 1½ cup serving.

Yield: 8 servings

Calories: 168
Exchanges: *1½ Bread*
           2   Veg

Cholesterol: *0   Mg*
SF: *<1 Gm*
Fat: *1   Gm*
Sodium: *215 Mg*
Dietary Fiber: *5   Gm*

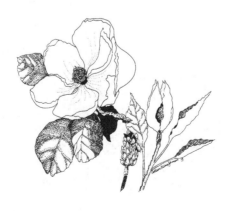

ELEGANT AMBROSIA COMPOTE

1	large can unsweetened pineapple
¼	cup sugar
1½	teaspoons pure apple juice
1	tablespoon lime juice
¼	teaspoon vanilla extract
1	sliced banana
3⅓	cups pineapple sherbet
8	ounces club soda

Drain pineapple, reserve ¼ cup juice. Combine reserved pineapple juice, sugar and next 3 ingredients. Stir until sugar dissolves. Set aside. Mix all fruit in a medium sized bowl. Pour juice over fruit and chill at least 4 hours or overnight. When ready to serve, spoon fruit mixture evenly into individual bowls or fruit cups. Top each serving with ⅓ cup sherbet and 2 tablespoons of club soda. Serve immediately. You may put entire fruit mixture into a pretty glass or crystal serving bowl. Serve immediately.

Yield: 8 (¾ cup) servings

Calories: 155
Exchanges: Not acceptable for diabetics.

Cholesterol:	*5*	*Mg*
SF:	*1*	*Gm*
Fat:	*2*	*Gm*
Sodium:	*35*	*Mg*
Dietary Fiber:	*3*	*Gm*

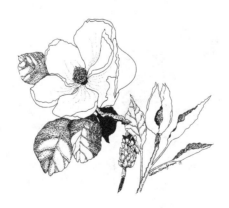

SPRINGTIME ASPARAGUS SALAD

1 pound fresh asparagus
¼ cup Italian fat free salad dressing
2 cups cooked macaroni
¾ cup fat free mayonnaise
2 tablespoons catsup
½ teaspoon prepared horseradish
½ teaspoon prepared mustard
2 chopped green onions
½ pound cooked, boneless, skinless chicken breast
1 cup diced celery

Put ¼ cup water into a 2 quart casserole. Add 1 pound fresh asparagus and microwave for 2 minutes. Drain well and marinate overnight in ¼ cup of fat free Italian dressing. Cook macaroni as directed, omitting any oil. Drain. Rinse with cold water. Drain again. Blend mayonnaise, catsup, horseradish, mustard and green onion. Mix together all ingredients.

Yield: 8 (1 cup) servings

Calories: 130
Exchanges: *1 Meat*
               1 Bread
               ½ Veg

Cholesterol: *22*
SF: *<1 Gm*
Fat: *1   Gm*
Sodium: *472 Mg*
Dietary Fiber: 1 Gm

CALICO MOLD

1 tablespoon dry gelatin
1 cup water
8 ounces fat free sour cream
8 ounces light grated cheddar cheese
1 can (4 ounces) chopped green chilies
2 tablespoons pimientos
2 tablespoons chopped ripe olives
1 tablespoon chopped onion
   vegetable cooking spray

Sprinkle gelatin over cold water. Let stand 3 to 4 minutes. Stir over low heat until it dissolves, set aside. Combine sour cream and cheddar cheese. Stir in pepper chilies, pimientos, olives and onion. Gradually stir in gelatin. Refrigerate until mixture mounds when dropped from a spoon (30 to 45 minutes). Stir and spoon into a 4 cup fluted mold sprayed with cooking spray.

Yield: 76 (1 tablespoon) servings

Calories: 12 per tablespoon
Exchanges: Free

Cholesterol: *2* *Mg*
SF: *<1* *Gm*
Fat: *<1* *Gm*
Sodium: *50* *Mg*
Dietary Fiber: *0* *Gm*

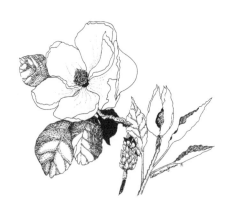

THREE BEAN SALAD

1   can (16 ounces) yellow wax beans, no salt added
1   can (16 ounces) kidney beans, no salt added
1   can (16 ounces) green beans, no salt added
1   medium purple onion, sliced
½   cup fat free mayonnaise
⅛   teaspoon black pepper

Open cans of beans. Drain. Slice onion. Mix all ingredients together. Allow to chill in refrigerator at least one hour. This is an excellent salad to serve with oven fried fish.

Yield: 12 servings

Calories: 60
Exchanges: *½ Bread*
                    1 Veg

Cholesterol: *0 Mg*
SF: *0 Gm*
Fat: *<1 Gm*
Sodium: *224 Mg*
Dietary Fiber: *3 Gm*

CHICKEN AND SNOW PEA SALAD

½   pound cooked chicken breasts, skinned and chopped
5   ounces raw macaroni
1   small package (6 ounces) snow peas
¼   cup fat free French dressing
1   cup cherry tomatoes, cut in half

Cook macaroni with fat or salt. Drain well. Steam pea pods about 2 - 4 minutes in microwave and drain well. Mix mayonnaise and fat free French dressing in large bowl. Add remaining ingredients and toss.

Yield: 4 servings

Calories: 309
Exchanges: *1½ Meat*
                    2 Bread
                    1 Veg

Cholesterol: *43 Mg*
SF: *<1 Gm*
Fat: *2 Gm*
Sodium: *413 Mg*
Dietary Fiber: *2 Gm*

CHILLED CHICKEN AND PASTA SALAD

1	pound boneless skinned chicken breasts
1	dehydrated chicken bouillon cube
2½	cups water
½	cup chopped onions
6	ounces raw spaghetti pasta
1	can artichoke hearts
1	large chopped tomato
1	tablespoon olive oil
3	tablespoon Balsamic vinegar
3	tablespoon lemon juice
1½	tablespoons sugar
	dash of salt
½	teaspoon dried rosemary
¼	teaspoon garlic powder
¼	teaspoon black pepper

Dissolve bouillon cube in water. Add chicken and onion and cook until done, about 25 - 30 minutes. Reserve broth Allow chicken to cool and chop into bite sized pieces. Cook pasta according to package directions in reserved broth plus enough water added to comply with the package directions. Omit any added fat. Combine all ingredients and mix well. Refrigerate at least 2 hours.

Yield: 8 servings

Calories: 223
Exchanges: 2 *Meat*
              1 *Bread*
              1 *Veg*

Cholesterol: 44 *Mg*
SF: 1 *Gm*
Fat: 4 *Gm*
Sodium: 215 *Mg*
Dietary Fiber: 6 *Gm*

OLD FASHIONED CHICKEN SALAD

4 cups chicken breast, skinned, cooked and chopped
4 egg whites
1 cup celery, diced
¼ cup onions, chopped
¼ teaspoon salt
   dash of white pepper
   dash of red pepper
2 tablespoons lemon juice
½ cup fat free mayonnaise

Combine the first 8 ingredients. Mix gently. Fold in mayonnaise. Cover and chill for 2 hours. Spoon into a serving dish. Sprinkle with paprika. Garnish with parsley and tomatoes. (White water packed tuna may be substituted in this recipe).

Yield: 32 appetizer servings

Calories: 28
Exchanges: *½ Meat*

Cholesterol: *11 Mg*
SF: *<1 Gm*
Fat: *<1 Gm*
Sodium: *82 Mg*
Dietary Fiber: <1 Gm

JACK'S POLKA DOT SALAD

6 cups cabbage, shredded
8 ounces pineapple tidbits in light syrup
4 ounces fat free cheddar cheese, shredded
¾ cup seedless raisins

Combine all ingredients in a large mixing bowl. Stir gently to mix. Chill 1 - 2 hours before serving.

Yield: 16 (½ cup) servings

Calories: 62
Exchanges: *½ Veg*

Cholesterol: *1 Mg*
SF: *0 Gm*
Fat: *0 Gm*
Sodium: *248 Mg*
Dietary Fiber: 1 Gm

CORN AND CUCUMBERS

2 cups sliced cucumbers
1 large white onion
1 can sweet corn
½ cup white vinegar
2 tablespoons water
2 tablespoons sugar, or 6 packages of Equal may be substituted
1 teaspoon dried dill weed
¼ teaspoon black pepper
⅛ teaspoon red pepper

Peel cucumbers. Slice onion and cucumbers into thin slices. Drain corn. Combine all other ingredients. Pour over cucumbers, onion and corn. Cover and chill.

Yield: 8 (½ cup) servings

Calories: 87 with sugar; 78 with Equal
Exchanges: *1   Bread*
               ½   Veg

Cholesterol: *0   Mg*
SF: *0   Gm*
Fat: *0   Gm*
Sodium: *169 Mg*
Dietary Fiber   *2   Gm*

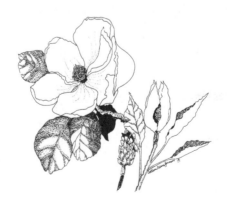

FRESH CORN SALAD

¼ cup fat free sour cream
¼ cup fat free mayonnaise
1 tablespoon vinegar (to taste)
1 tablespoon prepared yellow mustard
1 teaspoon sugar
¼ teaspoon salt
   dash of black pepper
2 cups boiled frozen corn kernels
2 ounces pimientos
½ cup diced raw carrots
½ cup chopped onions

Combine sour cream, mayonnaise, mustard, vinegar, sugar, salt and pepper. Add corn, pimientos, carrots and onion. Toss to blend. Cover and refrigerate at least one hour. It is even better to make this salad the day before.

Yield: 8 (½ cup) servings

Calories: 58
Exchanges: ½ *Bread*
             ½ *Veg*

Cholesterol: 0 *Mg*
SF: 0 *Gm*
Fat: 0 *Gm*
Sodium 199 *Mg*
Dietary Fiber: 2 *Gm*

FRUIT SALAD

1   can peach pie filling
1   small can Mandarin oranges, no sugar added
1   cup unsweetened sliced strawberries
4   bananas
1   large can unsweetened pineapple chunks

Thaw strawberries, slice bananas, drain pineapple and Mandarin oranges. Mix all ingredients together and chill in clear salad bowl.

Yield: 8 servings

Calories: 145
Exchanges: *2*   *Fruit*

Cholesterol: *0*   *Mg*
SF: *<1*   *Gm*
Fat: *<1*   *Gm*
Sodium: *#28 Mg*
Dietary Fiber: *2*   *Gm*

LIME JELLO SALAD

1   large box sugar free lime Jello
1   cup boiling water
1   cup evaporated skim milk
1   can fruit cocktail, no sugar added
1   cup fat free cottage cheese
¼   cup chopped pecans
½   tablespoon fat free mayonnaise

Mix Jello with hot water. Stir until dissolved. Cool. Stir in evaporated milk and add remaining ingredients. Put into a 9" x 13" pan. Chill. Serve in squares on lettuce leaves.

Yield: 12 servings

Calories: 52
Exchanges: *½*   *Fat*

Cholesterol: *2*   *Mg*
SF: *0*   *Gm*
Fat: *1*   *Gm*
Sodium: *447 Mg*
Dietary Fiber: *0*   *Gm*

MEXICAN SALAD

8	cups shredded lettuce
½	cup chopped onions
2	cups diced tomatoes
1	can (15 ounces) Healthy Valley vegetarian chili
4½	cups fat free cheddar cheese
1⅕	cups fat free Catalina salad dressing
16	ounces baked tortilla chips

Combine all ingredients in a large salad bowl and toss gently. Serve immediately.

Yield: 10 servings

Calories: 301
Exchanges: 1   *Meat*
               2   *Bread*
               2   *Veg*

Cholesterol: 5   *Mg*
SF: <1 *Gm*
Fat: 2   *Gm*
Sodium: 909 *Mg*
Dietary Fiber: 8   *Gm*

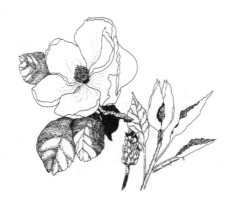

ENGLISH PEA SALAD

2 cups frozen petite English peas
½ cup shell pasta, dry
1 tablespoon chopped onion
1 hard boiled egg, chopped
1 cup shredded fat free cheddar cheese
3 tablespoons fat free mayonnaise

Drain peas. Cook and drain shell macaroni. Mix all ingredients together and chill before serving.

Yield: 6 (½ cup) servings

Calories: 121
Exchanges: *1   Meat*
               1   Bread

Cholesterol: *51 Mg*
SF: *<1 Gm*
Fat: *1   Gm*
Sodium: *291 Mg*
Dietary Fiber: *2   Gm*

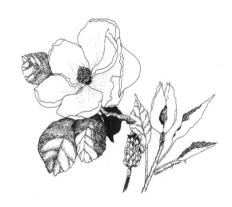

LOW CALORIE MANDARIN ORANGE SALAD

- 4 cups iceberg lettuce, chopped
- 4 cups Romaine lettuce, shredded
- 1 cup chopped mushrooms
- 1 cup purple onions, chopped
- 2 tablespoons canola oil
- 1 teaspoon yellow mustard
- 2 ounces balsamic vinegar
- ¼ cup water
- 2 small cans Mandarin oranges
- 24 packages (16 tablespoons) sugar substitute

Mix lettuce, mushrooms and purple onion in large bowl. Drain Mandarin oranges. Add to salad. Set aside. In a medium sized mixing bowl, mix sugar substitute, oil, mustard, vinegar, water and salt. Before serving salad, stir dressing and pour over salad and greens. Serve with grilled chicken, steamed broccoli with butter substitute and fresh French bread.

Yield: 6 servings

Calories: 115
Exchanges: *1* *Veg*
                 1 *Fruit*
                 1 *Fat*

Cholesterol: *0* *Mg*
SF: *<1* *Gm*
Fat: *5* *Gm*
Sodium: *114Mg*
Dietary Fiber: *2* *Gm*

EASY GERMAN POTATO SALAD

4   cups potatoes, boiled and cubed
1   cup onion, chopped
1   can (10 ounce) Healthy Request cream of chicken soup
¼   cup water
3   tablespoons vinegar
½   teaspoon sugar
   dash black pepper
1   teaspoon dried parsley
2   slices turkey bacon
1½ teaspoons liquid smoke
   vegetable cooking spray

You may cook the potatoes the night before by boiling in water with jackets on. Chill in the refrigerator overnight. Or, you may choose to bake the potatoes in the microwave.

Cook turkey bacon until crisp. Remove, drain and set aside. Spray skillet with cooking spray. Add onion. Cook until tender and transparent. Blend in soup, water, vinegar, sugar, liquid smoke and pepper. Heat. Stir occasionally for 2 - 3 minutes. Add potatoes, parsley and crisp, crumbled bacon.

Yield: 6 servings

Calories: 164
Exchanges: 2   Bread

Cholesterol: 4   Mg
SF: <1 Gm
Fat: 2   Gm
Sodium: 175 Mg
Dietary Fiber: 3   Gm

RED POTATO SALAD

  3 **pounds (approximately 10) red potatoes**
      olive oil flavored cooking spray
  1 **cup chopped green onions**
  ½ **cup fresh parsley**
  ¼ **cup canned chopped pimientos**
  ½ **cup fat free yogurt**
  3 **tablespoons white wine vinegar**
  1 **tablespoon Grey Poupon Dijon mustard**
  ¼ **teaspoon black pepper**
  ¼ **teaspoon red or cayenne pepper**
  ¼ **teaspoon ground tarragon**

Bring potatoes to a boil in Dutch oven covered with water. Partially cover and simmer 25 minutes or until tender. Drain, let cool.

Sauté onions until lightly browned. Cut potatoes (in skins) into ¼" slices. Combine yogurt, and remaining ingredients. Toss gently to coat potatoes well.

Yield: 8 (1 cup) servings

Calories: 168
Exchanges: *2*   *Bread*

Cholesterol: *0* *Mg*
SF: *0* *Gm*
Fat: *1* *Gm*
Sodium: *72* *Mg*
Dietary Fiber: *2* *Gm*

SEA SHELL SALAD

8 ounces raw shell pasta
1½ pounds peeled shrimp
1 bay leaf
2 tablespoons dehydrated onion flakes
¼ teaspoon red pepper
½ cup frozen sugar snap peas
8 ounces canned Mandarin sections
5 green onions
1 tablespoon grated Parmesan cheese
¼ cup fat free Italian dressing

Boil water. Add shrimp, bay leaf, onion flakes and cayenne pepper. Boil for approximately 4 minutes or until shrimp are pink. Cool shrimp and peel and devein. Cook pasta according to package directions, omitting any fat. Drain and rinse in cold water. Thaw sugar snap peas. Mix peas and onions with salad dressing. Add shrimp and toss to thoroughly to mix all ingredients. Sprinkle with Parmesan cheese and chill. Salad tastes best when allowed to come to room temperature before serving.

Yield: 8 servings

Calories: 235
Exchanges: *2   Meat*
                2   Bread
                1   Veg

Cholesterol: *130 Mg*
SF: *<1 Gm*
Fat: *3   Gm*
Sodium: *269 Mg*
Dietary Fiber: *2   Gm*

TURKEY DELIGHT

    4   cups water
    1   pound cooked turkey breast, skinned
   12   ounces dry linguini
    6   ounces sweet peas, frozen
    6   chopped green onions
    2   cups diced tomato
    2   tablespoons olive oil
    1   tablespoon parsley
    1   cup balsamic vinegar
   ½   teaspoon oregano
    1   teaspoon basil
   ¼   teaspoon garlic powder
   ½   teaspoon black pepper

Cut turkey into small cubes. Cook linguini according to package directions, but do not use oil. Draining pasta. Rinse with cold water. Drain again. Mix vinegar, oil and seasonings. Combine all ingredients. Mix well. Cover and chill for 2 hours. This can be done the day before and chilled overnight.

Yield: 10 servings

Calories: 232
Exchanges: *2   Meat*
                  2   Bread
                  1   Veg

Cholesterol: *6   Mg*
SF: *1   Gm*
Fat: *4   Gm*
Sodium: *174 Mg*
Dietary Fiber: *1   Gm*

SEVEN LAYER VEGETABLE SALAD

4   ounces fat free sour cream
½   cup fat free mayonnaise
1   tablespoon yellow mustard
½   teaspoon dried dill weed
¼   teaspoon garlic powder
4   chopped green onions
¼   cup diced celery
¼   cup chopped bell pepper
1   cup frozen green peas, boiled and drained
5   cups torn lettuce
4   ounces grated fat free cheddar cheese
4   ounces Healthy Choice baked ham, diced

Blend sour cream, mayonnaise, mustard and dill weed in a large bowl. Layer in order over dressing: onion, celery, bell pepper, peas, torn lettuce. Sprinkle with cheese and top with diced ham (Bacon bits may be used in lieu of diced ham). Cover and refrigerate overnight or for at least 4 hours. Toss just before serving.

Yield: 6 (1 cup) servings

Calories: 109
Exchanges: *1   Meat*
                 ½   Bread
                 ½   Veg

Cholesterol: *13   Mg*
SF: *<1   Gm*
Fat: *1   Gm*
Sodium: *630 Mg*
Dietary Fiber: *2   Gm*

Entrées

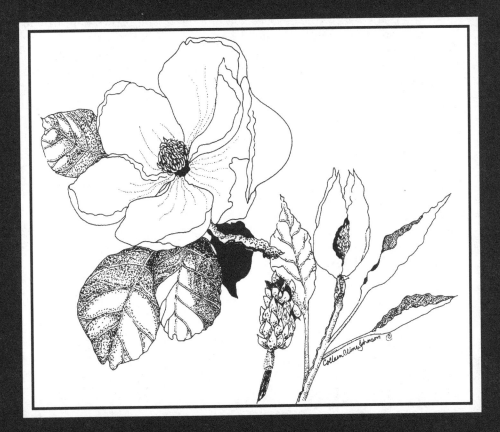

OVEN FRIED CATFISH

12   saltine crackers
½   cup skim milk
½   teaspoon dried parsley
1   teaspoon Louisiana hot sauce
    butter flavored cooking spray
1   pound catfish filets

Process saltines into fine cracker crumbs. Put cracker crumbs and parsley in a small bowl. Stir well. Mix hot sauce and milk in separate bowl. Dip filets in milk and hot sauce. Dredge through crumb mixture. Spray filets well with cooking spray. Bake uncovered at 400 degrees F for 20 - 25 minutes or until fish flakes easily when tested with a fork. Transfer to serving platter and serve immediately.

Yield: 4 servings

Calories: 161
Exchanges: *3*   *Meat*
               ½   *Bread*

Cholesterol: *66 Mg*
SF: *1*   *Gm*
Fat: *3*   *Gm*
Sodium: *183 Mg*
Dietary Fiber: *<1 Gm*

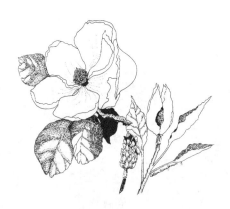

COURTBOUILLON

1 cup all purpose flour
1 cup onions, chopped
½ cup celery, chopped
½ cup bell peppers, chopped
4 cloves garlic
2 quarts water
¼ teaspoon salt
¼ teaspoon black pepper
¼ teaspoon red pepper
1 16 ounce can stewed tomatoes
olive oil flavored cooking spray
2½ pounds red snapper

Cut fish into 2" or 3" squares. (Any firm fish will do) Season with salt, black pepper and red pepper. Set aside. Spray a 5 quart or larger saucepan with vegetable cooking spray. Place over low heat. Add vegetables and cook for 40 minutes, uncovered. Mix 1 cup water with 1 cup flour. Add remaining water and flour mixture, bring to a boil, and cook an additional 30 minutes on low heat. Gently slip fish into sauce mixture and cook on medium heat uncovered another 30 minutes. Serve in large soup bowls or gumbo bowls with cooked rice and French bread.

Yield: 8 servings

Calories: 234
Exchanges: 4½ *Meat*
1 *Bread*
1½ *Veg*

Cholesterol: 52 *Mg*
SF: 1 *Gm*
Fat: 2 *Gm*
Sodium: 334 *Mg*
Dietary Fiber: 3 *Gm*

COURTBOUILLON (KOO-BEE-YON)

3 ribs chopped celery
2 cups chopped onion
1 cup fresh parsley
1 clove garlic
3 pounds catfish
¼ teaspoon salt
¼ teaspoon black pepper
¼ teaspoon red pepper
   vegetable cooking spray
2 tablespoons all purpose flour
1 can (8 ounces) tomato sauce
¼ cup water
¼ teaspoon ground thyme
2 bay leaves

Combine vegetables. Divide in half and set aside. Cut fish into large pieces, Generously sprinkle each piece with salt, pepper and red pepper. Set aside. Spray large saucepan with cooking spray. Add half of the fish in the bottom of the pan. Then, add half of the vegetables over the fish. Top with 1 tablespoon of flour, ¾ cup tomato sauce. Repeat layers one more time. Cover and cook over low heat for 1 hour or until the fish flakes easily. Shake pot occasionally to keep fish from sticking to the bottom of the pan. Do not stir as it will break up the fish.

Yield: 6 servings

Calories: 213
Exchanges: 5 *Meat*
                 1 *Bread*
                 ½ *Veg*

Cholesterol: 80 *Mg*
SF: 1   *Gm*
Fat: 2   *Gm*
Sodium: 176 *Mg*
Dietary Fiber: 1   *Gm*

CRAB AU GRATIN

1 cup chopped onions
6 chopped green onions
1 cup celery, diced
4 ounces dry butter substitute
4 tablespoons all purpose white flour
¼ teaspoon black pepper
8 ounces canned evaporated skim milk
1 cup skim milk
½ cup egg substitute
4 ounces light cheddar cheese
2 pounds fresh crab meat
vegetable cooking spray

Sauté onion and celery in butter substitute until soft. Add flour and blend well. Add milk and mix. Remove from heat. Add egg substitute, crab meat, salt, pepper and ¾ cup cheese. Mix well. Put in casserole prepared with cooking spray. Top with cheese. Bake at 350 degrees F until hot and cheese melts.

Yield: 8 (⅔ cup) servings

Calories: 206
Exchanges: 3 *Meat*
½ *Bread*
½ *Veg*
1 *Milk*

Cholesterol: 76 *Mg*
SF: 1 *Gm*
Fat: 3 *Gm*
Sodium: 791 *Mg*
Dietary Fiber: 1 *Gm*

CRAWFISH ETOUFFEE

2 pounds peeled crawfish
4 tablespoons dry substitute butter
½ cup chopped celery
1 cup chopped onions
¼ cup green onion tops
¼ cup bell pepper
1½ cups water
2 teaspoons cornstarch
¼ cup fresh parsley
¼ teaspoon black pepper
¼ teaspoon red pepper
¼ teaspoon salt
vegetable cooking spray

Sauté onion, pepper and celery in non-stick vegetable spray. Add water, crawfish, butter substitute and seasonings. Boil over low heat for 30 minutes. Add cornstarch mixed with 2 tablespoons of water. Add onion tops and parsley. Cook 10 minutes. Serve over rice.

Yield: 6 servings

Calories: 139
Exchanges: *3½ Meat*
                ½ Veg

Cholesterol: *173 Mg*
SF: *<1 Gm*
Fat: *2   Gm*
Sodium: *314 Mg*
Dietary Fiber: *1   Gm*

CRAWFISH PIE

1	teaspoon dry butter substitute
½	cup chopped onions
1	pound peeled crawfish tails
1	teaspoon seafood seasoning
¾	cup water
2	tablespoons cornstarch
5	green onions, chopped
10	sheets phyllo dough (sometimes called fillo dough)
¼	cup diced celery
	butter flavored cooking spray

Sauté onion and celery in butter flavored cooking spray. Add peeled crawfish tails. Cook 15 to 20 minutes. Add cornstarch and butter substitute that has been dissolved in water. Cook until thick. Add green onions and seasonings and mix well. Prepare pie plate with non-stick spray. Layer phyllo dough in a pie plate and with non-stick spray between each layer until all dough is used. Spray top of dough stack. Trim edges of dough around plate. Spray well. Pour filling (crawfish mixture) into pie crust and bake at 350 degrees F for 30 minutes. Let stand 5-10 minutes before cutting.

Yield: 6 servings

Calories: 169
Exchanges: *1½ Meat*
                   1½ Bread

Cholesterol: *81 Mg*
SF: *<1 Gm*
Fat: *3   Gm*
Sodium: *357 Mg*
Dietary Fiber: *<1 Gm*

CRAWFISH STEW

2 cups onion, chopped
1 cup diced celery
1 can (16 ounces) whole stewed tomatoes
4 cloves garlic
2 tablespoons tomato paste
1 cup fat free roux
10 chopped green onions
1 tablespoon chopped fresh parsley
1 gallon water
3 teaspoons seafood seasonings
2 pounds crawfish
   vegetable cooking spray

Scald crawfish. Put enough water in a heavy pot so that crawfish will be covered with about 4 inches of water. Bring to a boil. Drop crawfish into the boiling water. Turn off heat immediately. Allow crawfish to remain in hot water about 5 minutes in uncovered cooking pot. Drain and peel. (You may also buy crawfish already peeled and ready for use.) Prepare fat free roux. Refer to index for fat free roux. Spray large cooking pot with cooking spray. Heat to medium heat. Add onions, celery, whole tomatoes and tomato paste. Turn heat down and simmer about 30 minutes. Add fat free roux. Stir well to prevent lumping. Add gallon of hot water, garlic and seafood seasoning. Bring to a boil over high heat. Stir constantly. Lower heat and cook uncovered slowly for about 1 hour. Add crawfish tails and continue to cook slowly an additional 20 minutes. Add green onion tops and parsley. Serve with cooked rice, French bread and a large vegetable salad.

Yield: 12 servings

Calories: 123
Exchanges: *2*   *Meat*
              1   *Veg*

Cholesterol: *81 Mg*
SF: *<1 Gm*
Fat: *1   Gm*
Sodium: *531 Mg*
Dietary Fiber: *2   Gm*

BAKED FISH AU GRATIN

¼ diced cup celery
½ chopped cup onions
1 ounce dry substitute butter
½ teaspoon red pepper
¼ teaspoon black pepper
2 cups canned evaporated skim milk
1 ounce white sautérne
1½ pounds red snapper
½ pound shrimp, peeled and deveined
2 tablespoons bacon bits
3 tablespoons all purpose flour
½ cup bread crumbs

Spray skillet with cooking spray. Cook celery, onions over medium high heat until onions are wilted. Add flour, milk, butter substitute and black pepper. Stir constantly for 10 minutes or until thick. Add shrimp. Cook an additional 3 minutes. Add wine. Stir and remove from heat. Fish may be laid into individual or one large casserole that has been sprayed with cooking spray. Cook in a 350 degree F oven for 10 minutes. Pour sauce over fish and sprinkle with bread crumbs and bacon bits. Bake another 5 minutes or until crumbs brown.

Yield: 6 servings

Calories: 255
Exchanges: *4 Meat*
      1 Bread

Cholesterol: *102 Mg*
SF: *1 Gm*
Fat: *3 Gm*
Sodium: *345 Mg*
Dietary Fiber: *1 Gm*

GRILLED FISH POBOYS

4 poboy French bread buns
1 large tomato, sliced
4 tablespoons fat free mayonnaise
½ cup lettuce, shredded
4 tablespoons fat free Italian salad dressing
1 pound fish (red snapper, fresh tuna, amberjack, monk or Jew)

Marinate fish in fat free Italian salad dressing for 30 minutes.

Grill fish 3 to 4 minutes on each side. While filets are cooking, spray poboy buns with cooking spray and broil in the oven. Remove from oven. Spread buns with fat free mayonnaise. Add lettuce and tomatoes. Assemble and serve with new potatoes boiled in shrimp boil as a side dish.

Yield: 4 servings

Calories: 261
Exchanges: 3 *Meat*
2 *Bread*
½ *Veg*

Cholesterol: 41 *Mg*
SF: <1 *Gm*
Fat: 2 *Gm*
Sodium: 531 *Mg*
Dietary Fiber: 2 *Gm*

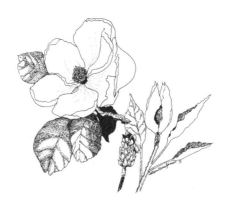

FLOUNDER AU GRATIN

¼ cup dry seasoned bread crumbs
2⅔ teaspoons grated Parmesan cheese
1 pound flounder filets (any fish may be substituted)
¼ cup fat free mayonnaise

Combine bread crumbs and cheese. Brush all sides of filets with mayonnaise. Roll coated filets in crumb mixture. Arrange in single layer in shallow baking sheet. Bake in preheated 375 degree F oven for 20 to 25 minutes or until fish flakes easily.

Yield: 4 servings

Calories: 151
Exchanges: 3 Meat
*   ½ Bread*

Cholesterol: 56 Mg
SF: <1 Gm
Fat: 2 Gm
Sodium: 509 Mg
Dietary Fiber: 0 Gm

STUFFED FLOUNDER

½ cup fat free salad dressing, French style
½ cup bread crumbs
¼ cup diced celery
4 green onions, cut up
1 pound flounder filets (any fish filet may be substituted)

Brush 2 tablespoons of fat free French dressing on the top side of fillets. In a measuring cup, combine ¼ cup dressing, bread crumbs, celery and onions. Divide into equal portions and place on fillets and roll up. You may secure with toothpick. Brush fillets with remaining dressing and bake at 350 degrees F for 35 minutes or until fish flakes when touched with fork.

Yield: 4 servings

Calories: 202
Exchanges: 3 Meat
*   1 Bread*

Cholesterol: 55 Mg
SF: <1 Gm
Fat: 2 Gm
Sodium: 736 Mg
Dietary Fiber: <1 Gm

OVEN FRIED OYSTERS

24 raw oysters
2 tablespoons all purpose flour
½ cup egg substitute
¼ cup water
dash of pepper
dash of salt
1 cup bread crumbs
vegetable cooking spray

Drain oysters and pat dry on a paper towel. Dredge each oyster in flour. In a shallow bowl, whisk together egg substitute, water, and seasonings. Dip each oyster in egg mixture, then in bread crumbs. Coat a large baking sheet with non-stick spray. Place oysters on the sheet and mist with non-stick spray. Bake at 450 degrees F until the coating becomes crisp.

Yield: 4 servings (6 oysters per serving)

Calories: 123
Exchanges: *1 Meat*
                      ½ Bread

Cholesterol: 46 Mg
SF: 1 Gm
Fat: 3 Gm
Sodium: 250 Mg
Dietary Fiber: <1 Gm

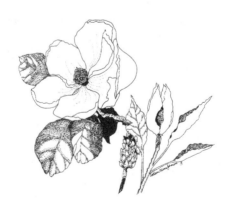

BAKED RED FISH

2 pounds red fish (any firm fish may be used)
1 cup onions, chopped
½ cup celery, diced
4 cloves garlic
4 ounces dry butter substitute
1 can (16 ounces) tomato sauce
1 can whole tomatoes
2 tablespoons lemon juice
2 cups water
¼ teaspoon black pepper
¼ teaspoon red pepper

Season fish with black and red pepper. Put into baking dish and set aside. Spray a skillet with cooking spray. Heat and add onion, celery and garlic. Cook until onions are wilted. Stir constantly. Add whole tomatoes and tomato sauce. Simmer about 30 minutes to blend flavors. Add 2 cups water Cook for 20 minutes. Pour mixture over fish in baking dish. Bake at 325 degrees F for 30 minutes. Spoon fish and sauce over rice. Serve with hot French bread and a green salad. Garnish with thin lemon slice if desired.

Yield: 6 servings

Calories: 198
Exchanges: *5*   *Meat*
              2   *Veg*

Cholesterol: *55 Mg*
SF: *1*   *Gm*
Fat: *3*   *Gm*
Sodium: *792 Mg*
Dietary Fiber: *2*   *Gm*

STUFFED RED SNAPPER

> 2 pounds red snapper fillets
> 1½ cups chopped onions
> ½ cup chopped celery
> olive oil flavored cooking spray
> ½ teaspoon sugar
> 1 teaspoon salt
> ¼ teaspoon red pepper
> ½ cup bread crumbs
> ¼ teaspoon black pepper
> 1 pound raw shrimp
> 6 ounces hamburger buns
> 1 cup egg substitute
> 2 tablespoons all purpose flour

STUFFING:

Boil shrimp, peel and chop in fairly large pieces. Spray skillet with cooking spray. Add onions and celery. Sauté until wilted. Add sugar, black pepper, salt and shrimp. Cook about 2 minutes. Put buns and egg beaters in a bowl. Mix well and add flour and bread crumbs. When well mixed, add shrimp mixture. Mix well.

FISH PREPARATION:

Make a slit (a pocket) in each fillet. Spray each fillet with cooking spray. Stuff each fillet with stuffing mixture. Broil in the oven 10 minutes on each side. Serve with liquid Butter Buds and lemon juice.

Yield: 8 servings

Calories: 248
Exchanges: *5   Meat*
               1   Bread
               1   Veg

Cholesterol: *115 Mg*
SF: *1   Gm*
Fat: *4   Gm*
Sodium: *545 Mg*
Dietary Fiber: *1   Gm*

PLANTATION SHRIMP WITH RICE

butter flavored cooking spray
2 pounds raw shrimp, peeled
¾ cup chopped onion
¼ cup green chopped onion
½ cup chopped bell pepper (red* or green)
1 pound sliced mushrooms
2 tablespoons liquid Butter Buds
1 tablespoon Worcestershire sauce
2 bay leaves
¼ teaspoon garlic powder
⅛ teaspoon black pepper
1 tablespoon parsley
2 cups cooked rice

Sauté onions, bell pepper and mushrooms in a skillet that has been sprayed with butter flavored cooking spray until vegetables are just tender. Stir in black pepper, garlic powder, liquid Butter Buds and bay leaves. Add shrimp and cook until shrimp turn pink. Mix in warm rice. Let sit for a few minutes before serving. Remove bay leaves. Sprinkle with parsley. *If you use the red bell pepper, it makes a nice holiday casserole.

Yield: 8 servings

Calories: 214
Exchanges: *3*   *Meat*
            1   *Bread*
            1   *Veg*

Cholesterol: *175 Mg*
SF: *< 1 Gm*
Fat: *2   Gm*
Sodium: *193 Mg*
Dietary Fiber: *1   Gm*

SEAFOOD LASAGNA

2 (10 ounce) packages raw spinach, chopped
½ cup all purpose flour
2 cups canned skim evaporated milk
⅛ teaspoon red pepper or cayenne
⅛ teaspoon black pepper
¼ teaspoon garlic powder
¼ cup white table wine
⅔ cup grated Parmesan cheese
1 pound raw, peeled shrimp
2 ounces whole fresh basil
½ pound raw crab meat
1 tablespoon lemon juice
9 lasagna noodles, cooked (8 ounces)
2 egg whites
½ teaspoon paprika

Press spinach between paper towels until dry. Set aside. Place flour in shallow pan. Bake for 30 minutes at 350 degrees F until lightly browned, stirring often. Spoon flour into large saucepan. Gradually add milk and blend with a wire whisk. Stir in the next 3 ingredients. Add wine and cook 1 minute. Remove from heat. Stir in shrimp, crab and ½ cup cheese. Reserve 1 cup sauce and add spinach, basil, lemon juice and egg whites. Spoon ¼ cup seafood sauce into a 13" x 9" x 2" baking dish. Arrange 3 lasagna noodles over sauce. Spoon ⅓ spinach mixture over noodles. Combine remaining cheese and paprika. Sprinkle over lasagna. Bake covered at 400 degrees F for 30 minutes. Bake uncovered 10 minutes. Let stand 10 - 15 minutes before serving.

Yield: 9 (3" x 4") servings

Calories: 280
Exchanges: 3   *Meat*
　　　　　　 2   *Bread*
　　　　　　 ½   *Veg*

Cholesterol: 11   *Mg*
SF: <1   *Gm*
Fat: 4   *Gm*
Sodium: 60   *Mg*
Dietary Fiber: 0   *Gm*

SHRIMP AND ANGEL HAIR PASTA

8 ounces raw, peeled shrimp
4 ounces angel hair pasta
4 fluid ounces liquid butter substitute
¾ cup skimmed evaporated milk
2 ounces chopped fresh parsley
½ teaspoon dried dill weed
2 cloves of garlic
dash of black pepper

Peel and devein shrimp. Set aside. Cook pasta according to package directions, eliminating oil. Drain and set aside. Cook butter substitute, shrimp and garlic over medium-high heat in a heavy skillet. Cook 3 to 5 minutes, stirring constantly. Remove shrimp and set aside. Reserve garlic and butter substitute mixture. Add evaporated skim milk mixed with 1 tablespoon cornstarch and cook on low until thicken, stirring constantly. Add shrimp, parsley and seasonings. Stir until blended. Serve over angel hair pasta.

Yield: 2 servings

Calories: 446
Exchanges: *3½ Meat*
          2 Bread
          ½ Milk

Cholesterol: *178 Mg*
SF: *<1 Gm*
Fat: *3 Gm*
Sodium: *850 Mg*
Dietary Fiber: *0 Gm*

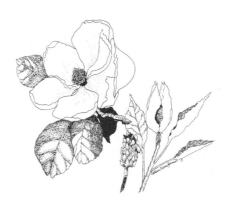

SHRIMP STUFFED BELL PEPPER

1	pound raw, peeled shrimp
½	cup celery, diced
½	cup onion, chopped
2	ounces dry butter substitute
1	cup cooked rice
5	ounces tomato paste
8	bell peppers
½	cup bread crumbs
1	clove garlic
¼	teaspoon black pepper
	olive oil flavored cooking spray
2⅔	tablespoons Parmesan cheese, grated

PEPPERS:

Cut off tops and remove centers of peppers. Put peppers into cold water and bring to a boil. Boil for 5 minutes. Drain, turn upside on a paper towel. Set aside.

STUFFING:

Spray saucepan with cooking spray. Add onions, celery and tomato paste. Let cook until onions are wilted. Add shrimp and cook an additional 4 minutes or until shrimp turn pink. Add rice, butter substitute and seasonings. Mix well. Stuff each pepper with stuffing. Sprinkle with bread crumbs. Spray each pepper top with cooking spray and top with 1 teaspoon Parmesan cheese. Bake at 350 degrees F for 15 minutes.

Yield: 8 servings

Calories: 144
Exchanges: 2 *Meat*
              ½ *Bread*
              2 *Veg*

Cholesterol: 88 *Mg*
SF: 1 *Gm*
Fat: 2 *Gm*
Sodium: 236 *Mg*
Dietary Fiber: 2 *Gm*

SHRIMP CREOLE

vegetable cooking spray
12 ounces raw shrimp, peeled
¼ cup all purpose flour
¼ teaspoon red pepper
6 ounces tomato paste
½ cup bell pepper, chopped
1½ cups water
¼ teaspoon salt
1 tablespoon crumbled bay leaf
2 cloves garlic
1 cup chopped onion
2 tablespoons parsley
¼ cup green onion, chopped
2 cups cooked rice

Brown flour in skillet by constantly stirring until a caramel color. Do not over-cook or it will have a burned taste. Set aside. Place garlic, onion, parsley and bell pepper in another (heavy) skillet that has been sprayed with vegetable cooking spray. Cook vegetables until tender. Add 1 cup of water. Add all remaining ingredients except the shrimp, browned flour and ½ cup of water. Cook on high heat. Bring to a boil. Reduce heat Add browned flour to the remaining ½ cup of water. Mix well to make a paste. Gradually add the browned flour paste to the vegetables. Add shrimp. Stir well over low heat. Simmer Creole for 20 to 30 minutes covered. Serve over rice.

Yield: 4 (1 cup Creole plus ½ cup rice) servings

Calories: 290
Exchanges: *3*   *Meat*
            2   *Bread*
            2   *Veg*

Cholesterol: *131 Mg*
SF: *<1 Gm*
Fat: *2 Gm*
Sodium: *395 Mg*
Dietary Fiber: *4 Gm*

SHRIMP WITH EGGPLANT CASSEROLE

- **16** ounces raw shrimp
- **1** large eggplant
- **1** cup chopped onion
- **1** cup chopped bell pepper
- **1** cup chopped celery
- **10** ounces Campbell's Healthy Request cream of mushroom soup
- **½** teaspoon black pepper
- **1** clove garlic
- **4** ounces light cheddar cheese
- **½** cup dry seasoned bread crumbs

Puncture eggplant several times and cook on high in microwave for 3 minutes. Set aside to cool. When cool pull skin off and chop. Sauté shrimp, onion, bell pepper, celery and garlic in cooking spray until the shrimp turn pink. Add soup and cheese, heat and set aside. Mix with ¼ cup seasoned bread crumbs and chopped eggplant. Top with remaining bread crumbs and spray with cooking spray. Bake at 350 degrees F for 25 minutes.

Yield: 8 servings

Calories: 162
Exchanges:

	2	*Meat*
	½	*Bread*
	1	*Veg*
	½	*Fat*

Cholesterol:	*94*	*Mg*
SF:	*1*	*Gm*
Fat:	*4*	*Gm*
Sodium:	*562*	*Mg*
Dietary Fiber:	*1*	*Gm*

SHRIMP AND OKRA CREOLE

2 pounds raw shrimp, peeled
3 quarts water
1 tablespoon tomato paste
1 pound okra, cut up
1 cup onions, chopped
½ cup diced celery
½ cup chopped bell pepper
1 cup fresh peeled tomato, chopped
4 cloves garlic
½ teaspoon salt
⅓ teaspoon red pepper
   olive oil flavored cooking spray
1 tablespoon dry butter substitute
8 green onions
¼ cup parsley

Spray large cooking pot or saucepan with cooking spray. Cook okra, tomato paste, fresh tomato, onions, garlic, celery and bell pepper about 30 minutes over low heat. Add water and season to taste. Cook for 45 - 60 minutes. Add shrimp. Cook an additional 20 minutes. Add green onion tops and parsley 5 minutes before serving. Serve over cooked rice.

Yield: 8 servings

Calories: 219
Exchanges: 4   *Meat*
                2   *Veg*

Cholesterol: 230 *Mg*
SF: 1   *Gm*
Fat: 3   *Gm*
Sodium: 485 *Mg*
Dietary Fiber: 1   *Gm*

CHEESY SHRIMP NOODLE BAKE

16 ounces raw shrimp
 7 ounces raw pasta noodles
 8 ounces fat free sour cream
½ cup chopped onions
 2 olives, sliced
 1 teaspoon dried dill weed
 4 ounces low fat cheddar cheese
10 ounces Campbell's Healthy Request cream of
     mushroom soup

Combine noodles, sour cream, soup, onions, olives, seasoning and half the cheese. Mix until well blended and fold in shrimp. Spoon into shallow baking dish. Top with other half of cheese. Bake at 350 degrees F for 30 to 35 minutes.

Yield: 8 servings

Calories: 214
Exchanges: *3   Meat*
                 1   Bread

Cholesterol: *94 Mg*
SF: *1   Gm*
Fat: *4   Gm*
Sodium: *363 Mg*
Dietary Fiber: *0   Gm*

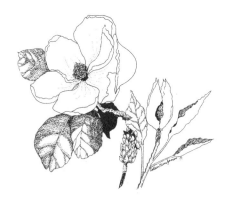

TUNA CASSEROLE

1   can Healthy Request cream of mushroom soup
1⅓ cups water
¼   cup chopped onions
1   teaspoon lemon juice
¼   teaspoon salt
    dash black pepper
1⅓ cups instant white rice
10 ounces frozen green beans
1   7 ounce can water packed tuna fish
2   ounces light cheddar cheese
    vegetable cooking spray

Combine water, soup, onion, lemon juice, salt and pepper in a saucepan. Bring mixture to boil. Pour half of the mixture into a 1½ quart casserole that has been sprayed with cooking spray. Layer other ingredients as follows: rice, peas, tuna and remaining soup mixture. Sprinkle with cheese. Cover and bake at 375 degrees F for 10 minutes. Stir, cover and cook an additional 15 minutes.

Yield: 4 (1⅓ cup) servings

Calories: 296
Exchanges: 2   *Meat*
              2   *Bread*

Cholesterol: 42 *Mg*
SF: 1   *Gm*
Fat: 3   *Gm*
Sodium: 712 *Mg*
Dietary Fiber: 3   *Gm*

CHICKEN AND ASPARAGUS

1½	pounds chicken breasts, skinned
1	cup diced onion
1	cup chopped mushrooms
1	16 ounce package frozen asparagus
1	10 ounce can Healthy Request cream of mushroom soup
6	ounces evaporated skim milk
½	cup fat free cheddar cheese, grated
¼	teaspoon Tabasco sauce
¼	teaspoon black pepper
1	tablespoon Kikkoman lite soy sauce
2	tablespoons canned pimiento
1	ounce chopped almonds

Boil chicken and cut into bite sized pieces. Set aside. Place in the bottom of a 13" x 9" pan a layer of asparagus and then chicken pieces. In a large skillet, sauté onions and mushrooms for about 2 minutes. Add soup, milk, cheese, Tabasco, soy sauce, salt and pimiento. Simmer mixture until cheese melts, stirring constantly (fat free cheeses have a tendency to scorch easily). Pour over chicken and bake for 20-25 minutes at 350 degrees F until bubbly. Top with almonds.

Yield: 8 servings

Calories: 224
Exchanges: 4   *Meat*
              1   *Veg*

Cholesterol: 69 *Mg*
SF: 1 *Gm*
Fat: 5 *Gm*
Sodium: 328 *Mg*
Dietary Fiber: 1 *Gm*

CHICKEN ASPARAGUS FETTUCCINI

    vegetable cooking spray
½ cup skim evaporated milk
¾ cup chopped mushrooms
1 cup chopped onions
12 ounces frozen asparagus
8 ounces raw fettuccini noodles
¾ tablespoon dried parsley
    dash black pepper
8 ounces cooked, cubed chicken breast
4 ounces low fat cheddar cheese
1 can Healthy Request cream of chicken soup

Cook fettuccini by package directions, omitting any fat. Drain. Wash and drain fresh asparagus well and cut each stalk in 3 pieces. Combine chicken, fettuccini and asparagus. Heat soup with skim evaporated milk. Add onions, mushrooms, parsley and pepper. Pour over chicken mixture and toss. Place in casserole pan prepared with vegetable cooking spray. Top with cheese. Heat in 350 degree oven until cheese melts.

Yield: 8 servings

Calories: 259
Exchanges: *1½ Meat*
                1½ Bread
                ½ Veg

Cholesterol: *65 Mg*
SF: *1 Gm*
Fat: *6 Gm*
Sodium: *307 Mg*
Dietary Fiber: *1 Gm*

QUICK CHICKEN AND DUMPLINGS

8 ounces boneless, skinless chicken breast
2 tablespoons dry butter substitute
   dash black pepper
¼ cup diced celery
¼ chopped onions
10 fat free tortillas
1 cube chicken bouillon
5 cups water

Cook chicken breasts in a large pot filled with 5 cups water, 1 bouillon cube, onion and celery. Cook until tender. Remove chicken. Cut into bite sized pieces. Cut fat free flour tortillas into strips. Bring broth to a boil. Add butter substitute. Drop strips in boiling broth mixture. Cook about 10 - 12 minutes. Add chicken. Pepper to taste.

Yield: 8 servings

Calories: 169
Exchanges: *1*   *Meat*
                 2   *Bread*

Cholesterol: 22   *Mg*
SF: 1   *Gm*
Fat: 2   *Gm*
Sodium: 561   *Mg*
Dietary Fiber: <1   *Gm*

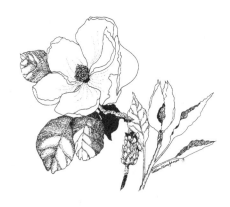

CHICKEN AND PASTA

8 ounces pasta
½ cups broccoli
½ cups carrot, shredded
2 green onions
½ bell peppers, chopped
1 can Healthy Request mushroom soup
¾ cup water
½ cup Parmesan cheese, grated
8 ounces cooked, skinned, chicken
1 tablespoon seafood seasoning

Cook pasta according to package directions, but with no oil. While pasta is cooking, add all vegetables the last 5 minutes of cooking time. Drain. Heat cheese, water and soup. Combine pasta, vegetables and chicken with soup mixture. Cook over low heat for 5 - 8 minutes.

Yield: 8 servings

Calories: 188
Exchanges: *1 Meat*
             1 Bread
             1 Veg

Cholesterol: *27 Mg*
SF: *3 Gm*
Fat: *2 Gm*
Sodium: *239 Mg*
Dietary Fiber: *1 Gm*

CHICKEN AND RICE

4 chicken breasts, skinned
½ cup liquid Butter Buds
1 cup long grain rice, uncooked
2 green onions, chopped
6 ounces Healthy Request cream of mushroom soup
1 tablespoon Worcestershire sauce
¼ teaspoon black pepper

Sprinkle chicken breasts with black pepper. Mix butter substitute, rice, onion, soup and Worcestershire sauce in casserole dish. Place chicken on top of this mixture. Cover with aluminum foil with holes punched in top. Bake at 350 degrees F for 1½ hours.

Yield: 4 servings

Calories: 330
Exchanges: *4*   *Meat*
                2   *Bread*

Cholesterol: *70 Mg*
SF: *1*   *Gm*
Fat: *4*   *Gm*
Sodium: *540 Mg*
Dietary Fiber: *1*   *Gm*

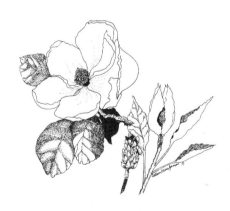

CHICKEN STIR-FRY AND BROWN RICE

3 ounces chopped Canadian bacon
½ cup chopped onions
12 ounces boneless, skinless chicken, cubed
4 ounces canned mushrooms, drained
3 cups cooked rice
¼ cup sliced pimientos
   dash of black pepper
2 tablespoons low salt soy sauce
1 cup snow peas

In a large skillet, sauté chopped Canadian bacon and onions until onions are transparent. Add chicken and cook 5-10 minutes until chicken is slightly brown and done. Stir in remaining ingredients. Heat thoroughly.

Yield: 6 servings

Calories: 309
Exchanges: 3   *Meat*
            1½ Bread
            2   *Veg*

Cholesterol: 37 *Mg*
SF: 2   *Gm*
Fat: 4   *Gm*
Sodium: 702 *Mg*
Dietary Fiber: 5   *Gm*

CHICKEN AND YELLOW RICE

 3 pounds skinless chicken breasts
16 ounces diced canned tomatoes
 1 cup chopped onion
 1 cup chopped bell pepper
 2 cloves garlic
 2 cups white long grain rice
 3 bay leaves
48 ounces defatted chicken broth
 2 teaspoons turmeric
 2 cups frozen English (tiny green) peas
    vegetable cooking spray

Cover the rice with water and soak overnight. Boil chicken and cut into bite size pieces. (This also may be done the night before). The next day, place chicken in large Dutch oven. Pour can of tomato pieces over the chicken. Meanwhile sauté vegetables in cooking spray. Add to chicken. Drain rice and add to chicken. Add bay leaves, broth and turmeric. Bake in 350 degree F oven for 20 minutes with lid off and 20 minutes with lid on. Add English peas and cook 5 minutes longer with lid on.

Yield: 12 servings

Calories: 341
Exchanges: *4   Meat*
                 2   Bread
                 1   Veg

Cholesterol: *87 Mg*
SF: *1   Gm*
Fat: *4   Gm*
Sodium: *253 Mg*
Dietary Fiber: *3   Gm*

CHICKEN AND SUN-DRIED TOMATO SAUCE

1 **pound skinless, boneless chicken, cut in strips**
½ **cup fat free chicken broth**
2 **ounces tomato slices sun dried (not oil packed)**
½ **cup raw mushrooms, sliced**
1 **green onion, chopped**
2 **cloves garlic**
2 **tablespoons red table wine**
   vegetable cooking spray
4 **ounces fettuccine, raw**
½ **cup skim milk**
2 **teaspoons cornstarch**
2 **teaspoons chopped basil**

Mix tomatoes with broth. Let stand 30 minutes. Cook chicken in skillet sprayed with cooking spray until brown on both sides. Remove and set aside. Add mushrooms, onions, garlic and wine. Cook on medium heat until mushrooms are tender. Add tomato mixture. Heat until boiling. Cover and simmer 10 minutes, stirring occasionally. Add milk, cornstarch and basil to tomato mixture. Boil and stir 1 minute. Serve over fettuccine prepared according to package directions, without adding fat or salt.

Yield: 4 servings

Calories: 323
Exchanges: *4*   *Meat*
           1   *Bread*
           ½   *Veg*

Cholesterol: *93*   *Mg*
SF: *1*   *Gm*
Fat: *5*   *Gm*
Sodium: *114* *Mg*
Dietary Fiber: *1*   *Gm*

COUNTRY BAKED CHICKEN

24 ounces chicken breasts, skinned and deboned
1 cup chopped mushrooms
1 cup diced celery
1 cup white table wine
½ cup sliced raw carrots
½ cup chopped onion
1 clove garlic
1 bay leaf
1 teaspoon dried parsley
¼ teaspoon ground thyme

Preheat oven to 350 degrees F. Line a 2 quart casserole with aluminum foil. Lay chicken breasts upon foil. Sprinkle chicken with seasonings and vegetables. Pour wine over entire mixture. Seal the foil tightly. Place in a 350 degree F oven. Bake for 35 - 45 minutes.

This dish is delicious with creamed new potatoes.

Yield: 6 (4 ounce) servings

Calories: 215
Exchanges: 4 *Meat*
1 *Veg*

Cholesterol: 87 *Mg*
SF: 1 *Gm*
Fat: 4 *Gm*
Sodium: 95 *Mg*
Dietary Fiber: 1 *Gm*

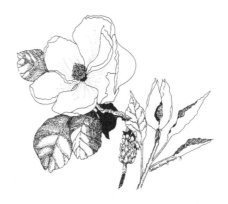

CAJUN FRENCH CHICKEN

1   **pound skinless chicken breast**
½   **cup fat free Kraft Catalina dressing**
1   **16 ounce can diced tomatoes**
1   **cup chopped onion**
1   **cup diced celery**
⅛   **teaspoon black pepper**
⅛   **teaspoon red pepper**
2   **ounces red wine**
2   **tablespoons all purpose flour**
    vegetable cooking spray

Pour ¼ cup salad dressing into skillet sprayed with cooking spray. Add chicken and brown over low heat. Add ¼ cup of dressing, tomatoes, onions, celery and seasonings. Cover and simmer for 20 minutes. Remove chicken and vegetables to serving platter, retaining liquid in skillet. In a cup gradually add wine to flour, stirring until well blended. Pour wine mixture in skillet containing hot liquid. Cook until mixture thickens, stirring constantly. Serve with rice.

Yield: 4 servings

Calories: 292
Exchanges: *4   Meat*
               ½   Bread
               2   Veg

Cholesterol: *96 Mg*
SF: *1   Gm*
Fat: *4   Gm*
Sodium: *734 Mg*
Dietary Fiber: *4   Gm*

CHICKEN DIVAN

2   10 ounce packages frozen broccoli spears, cooked and drained
12   ounces cooked chicken breast, skinned and sliced
2   cans Healthy Request cream of chicken soup
1   teaspoon lemon juice
2   ounces fat free cheddar cheese, grated
½   cup bread crumbs
1   tablespoon dry butter substitute

Place broccoli in 2 quart casserole. Layer chicken over broccoli. Mix soup, lemon juice and cheese together. Spread over chicken. Combine bread crumbs with butter buds. Toast until light brown and dry. Sprinkle crumbs evenly over top of casserole. Cook in microwave oven for 8 minutes on full power or until bubbly.

Yield: 6 servings

Calories: 152
Exchanges: *3*   *Meat*
                ½   *Bread*
                1   *Veg*

Cholesterol: *47*   *Mg*
SF: *1*   *Gm*
Fat: *3*   *Gm*
Sodium: *292*   *Mg*
Dietary Fiber: *3*   *Gm*

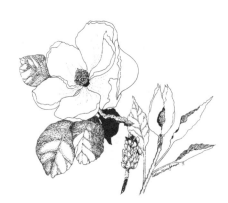

HAWAIIAN CHICKEN KABOBS

1½   pounds chicken breast, skinned, cooked and cubed
1   can (15¼ ounces) pineapple chunks packed in water
¼   cup lite soy sauce
1   ounce liquid Butter Buds
1   tablespoon brown sugar
1   teaspoon brown sugar
1   teaspoon garlic powder
2   teaspoons ground ginger
1   teaspoon black pepper
1   cup bell pepper chopped
12   mushrooms
1   cup tomato diced
3   cups water
1   cup long grain raw rice

Bring 3 cups of water to a boil in a saucepan. Add 1 cup raw rice. Stir, cover and cook for 20 minutes. When rice is done, rinse and set aside. While rice is cooking, place chicken cubes in large shallow container. Drain pineapple, reserving ½ cup of liquid. Set pineapple chunks aside. Combine liquid and the next 7 ingredients in a small saucepan to use as a marinade. Stir well. Bring to a boil. Reduce heat and simmer uncovered for 5 minutes. Pour over chicken. Cover and refrigerate at least 1 hour. Stir occasionally. Remove chicken from marinade. Reserve marinade. Alternate chicken, pineapple, bell pepper, tomato and mushrooms on skewers. Grill kabobs over hot coals for 20 minutes or until chicken is done. Baste with marinade frequently. Turn occasionally. Serve over cooked rice. This is a complete meal.

Yield: 6 (with ½ cup rice) servings

Calories: 349
Exchanges: *4*   *Meat*
              1   *Bread*
              1   *Veg*
              1   *Fruit*

Cholesterol: *87*   *Mg*
SF: *1*   *Gm*
Fat: *4*   *Gm*
Sodium: *573*   *Mg*
Dietary Fiber: *2*   *Gm*

OVEN FRIED CHICKEN

½ **cup egg substitute**
1 **cup all purpose flour**
½ **cup skim milk**
   dash black pepper
   dash salt
   vegetable cooking spray
1 **pound chicken breast, skinned and deboned**

Mix egg substitute and milk. Set aside. Place flour and seasonings in a zip lock plastic bag. Dredge chicken breasts through egg mixture then through flour mixture. Dip chicken in egg mixture and in the flour mixture again. Place on a baking pan that has been prepared with cooking spray. Spray each piece of chicken with cooking spray generously. Bake in 400 degree F oven for 25 minutes or until done.

Yield: 4 servings

Calories: 273
Exchanges: *4* *Meat*
             2 *Bread*

Cholesterol: *70* *Mg*
SF: *1* *Gm*
Fat: *3* *Gm*
Sodium: *173* *Mg*
Dietary Fiber: *1* *Gm*

HONEY GLAZED CHICKEN

1 tablespoons lite sauce soy sauce
3 tablespoons honey
½ teaspoon garlic powder
1 teaspoon yellow mustard
2 tablespoons lemon juice
½ teaspoon ginger
¼ teaspoon black pepper
2 pounds chicken breast, skinned

Combine all ingredients except chicken. Stir well. Set sauce aside. Grill chicken over medium coals. After turning chicken once, begin to baste with sauce until done.

Yield: 8 servings

Calories: 203
Exchanges: 4   *Meat*
                 ½   *Fruit*

Cholesterol: 87 *Mg*
SF: 1   *Gm*
Fat: 3   *Gm*
Sodium: 343 *Mg*
Dietary Fiber: <1 *Gm*

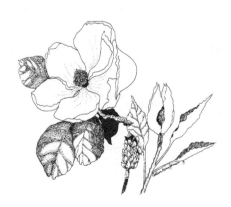

LOUISIANA CHICKEN JAMBALAYA

1 pound skinned chicken breast, cut in bite size pieces
1 pound Healthy Choice ground beef
2 cups white onions, chopped
1 cup chopped celery
3 cloves garlic
1 tablespoon tomato paste
3 cups cooked rice
5 green onions tops, chopped
½ teaspoon salt
½ teaspoon pepper
½ teaspoon parsley, chopped
   dash of red pepper
   vegetable cooking spray

Heat large Dutch oven that has been sprayed with vegetable cooking spray. Add onions, celery, garlic and tomato paste. Cook over medium heat uncovered until white onions are wilted. Add meats, salt, pepper and red pepper. Stir well until the meat starts to brown. Add one cup of cold water and continue to cook an additional 40 minutes on low heat. Stir occasionally. Add green onion tops and parsley. Simmer over low heat uncovered for an additional 15 minutes. Remove from heat. Add cooked rice and mix thoroughly. Serve with French bread and salad.

Yield: 8 servings

Calories: 248
Exchanges: 3 *Meat*
             1 *Bread*
             1 *Veg*

Cholesterol: 72 *Mg*
SF: 1 *Gm*
Fat: 4 *Gm*
Sodium: 332 *Mg*
Dietary Fiber: 1 *Gm*

SESAME CHICKEN KABOBS

1   pound cubed and skinned raw chicken breast
1   cup light soy sauce
¼   cup fat free salad dressing
1   teaspoon sesame seeds
2   tablespoons lemon juice
¼   teaspoon garlic powder
¼   teaspoon ground ginger
½   cup bell peppers
1   large onion
1½ cups sliced zucchini squash
2   cups diced tomatoes

Place chicken cubes in a large shallow container. Combine soy sauce, salad dressing, sesame seeds, juice, garlic powder and ginger in a jar. Cover tightly and shake vigorously to mix. Pour over chicken. Cover and refrigerate at least 2 hours. Stir chicken occasionally. Remove from marinade and reserve marinade. Alternate chicken and vegetables on skewers. Grill kabobs over medium-hot coals for 15 to 20 minutes or until chicken is done. Turn and baste frequently with marinade. Serve kabobs over a bed of wild rice.

Yield: 6 servings

Calories: 181
Exchanges: *2* *Meat*
             2 *Veg*

Cholesterol: *58 Mg*
SF: *<1 Gm*
Fat: *3 Gm*
Sodium: *615 Mg*
Dietary Fiber: *2 Gm*

LITE KING RANCH CHICKEN

4   4 ounce skinned, boneless chicken breasts
1   cup chopped onion
6   corn tortillas
½   cup fat free chicken broth
1   can Healthy Request cream of mushroom soup
1   can Healthy Request cream of chicken soup
½   cup tomatoes with green chilies
    vegetable cooking spray
2   cups fat free cheddar cheese

Boil and dice chicken. Combine soups, chicken, chicken broth, tomatoes and onion in saucepan on low heat until thoroughly mixed. In a casserole dish prepared with non-stick vegetable spray, alternate layers of tortillas and sauce mixture and cheese. Top with cheese. Bake at 350 degrees F for 20 to 25 minutes, until completely heated.

Yield: 8 servings

Calories: 171
Exchanges: *3*   *Meat*
             1   *Bread*
             ½   *Veg*

Cholesterol: *43* *Mg*
SF: *1*   *Gm*
Fat: *3*   *Gm*
Sodium: *419* *Mg*
Dietary Fiber: *0*   *Gm*

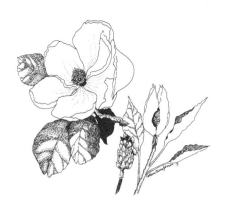

HOT CHICKEN SALAD

SALAD:

2   cups cubed, boneless, skinned, cooked chicken
½   cup diced celery
1   green chopped onion
¼   cup light cheddar cheese, grated
2   servings Mr. Phipp's Tator Crisps
    vegetable cooking spray

DRESSING:

1½   cups fat free mayonnaise
     dash of black pepper
1   tablespoon lemon juice
    dash of red pepper
¼   teaspoon salt

Combine dressing ingredients in a small bowl. Set aside. Combine chicken, celery, onion and cheese. Pour dressing over the salad ingredients. Place in casserole dish prepared with vegetable cooking spray. Top with crushed Tator Chips. Bake at 350 degrees F for 20 to 25 minutes.

Yield: 8 servings

Calories: 138
Exchanges: 2   Meat

Cholesterol: 36   Mg
SF: 1   Gm
Fat: 3   Gm
Sodium: 816 Mg
Dietary Fiber: <1 Gm

NEW ORLEANS STYLE CHICKEN

24	ounces skinned chicken breast, thinly sliced
	vegetable cooking spray
2	tablespoons all purpose flour
1	cup chopped onion
2	bell peppers, sliced in strips
16	ounces fat free chicken broth
20	ounces canned whole tomatoes
12	medium shrimp, peeled and deveined
6	raw oysters
2	tablespoons parsley
1	cup chopped raw mushrooms
1	cup white table wine

Sauté chicken in vegetable cooking spray. Remove chicken. Spray pan with cooking spray. Add bell pepper and onion. Sauté for 10 minutes. Add flour, chicken broth and tomatoes. Cook 5 minutes and return chicken strips to the pan. Add oysters, shrimp, parsley and mushrooms. Cook 15 minutes longer. Blend in wine and remove from heat.

Yield: 8 servings

Calories: 213
Exchanges: *4*   *Meat*
              1   *Veg*

Cholesterol: *98*   *Mg*
SF: *1*   *Gm*
Fat: *4*   *Gm*
Sodium: *287* *Mg*
Dietary Fiber: *1*   *Gm*

CHICKEN PAPRIKA

24 ounces chicken breast strips, boneless, skinless
⅓ cup all purpose flour
    vegetable cooking spray
2 cans (21 ounces) fat free tomato soup
½ cup water
1 cup mushrooms, sliced
½ cup chopped onions
1 teaspoon paprika
1 bay leaf
8 ounces fat free sour cream

Roll chicken in flour. Spray skillet with cooking spray and heat. Add chicken and cook until brown. Stir in remaining ingredients except sour cream. Cover. Simmer 45 minutes or until tender. Stir occasionally. Remove bay leaf. Blend in sour cream. Heat. Serve with noodles.

Yield: 8 servings

Calories: 188
Exchanges: *3* *Meat*
              1 *Bread*
              1 *Veg*

Cholesterol: *65 Mg*
SF: *1 Gm*
Fat: *3 Gm*
Sodium: *171 Mg*
Dietary Fiber: 2 Gm

FLAKEY CHICKEN PIE

1 pound skinless chicken breast
5 cups water
1 cup chopped onion
½ cup diced celery
1 bay leaf
17 ounces phyllo dough
¼ cup dry butter substitute
⅓ cup all purpose flour
¾ cup egg substitute
¼ cup fat free Parmesan cheese
¼ teaspoon white pepper
¼ teaspoon black pepper
5 ounces frozen peas and carrots
   vegetable cooking spray

Preheat oven to 350 degrees F. Combine first 5 ingredients in a Dutch oven. Bring to a boil. Cover and simmer on low heat for 30 minutes. Remove chicken and cool slightly. Cut chicken into bite size pieces. Set broth mixture to the side and remove bay leaf. Allow broth to cool to room temperature. Blend ½ cup of broth and flour. Stir until smooth. Add 2½ cups broth and egg substitute. Add cheese and peppers. Cook over low heat until thickened. Add chicken and set aside. Unfold phyllo (fillo) dough. Cut the stack of sheets in half crosswise. Trim each half to fit a 13" x 9" pan. Cover with damp dish towel. This will prevent dough from drying out. Coat bottom and sides with cooking spray. Lay 15 phyllo sheets in pan. Spray each layer with vegetable cooking spray. Spread half the chicken mixture over the phyllo. Top mixture with remaining trimmed phyllo sheets, spraying each sheet with cooking spray. Bake in preheated 350 degree F oven for 35 minutes.

Yield: 8 servings

Calories: 320
Exchanges: *2*   *Meat*
            1   *Veg*

Cholesterol: *51 Mg*
SF: *1*   *Gm*
Fat: *6*   *Gm*
Sodium: *424 Mg*
Dietary Fiber: *1*   *Gm*

POTLUCK CHICKEN

1	pound chicken breast, skinned
1½	pounds potatoes, quartered
1	cup fat free Parmesan cheese
1½	teaspoons garlic powder
16	ounces stewed tomatoes
2	teaspoons oregano
1	teaspoon black pepper
	olive oil flavored cooking spray

Place dry ingredients in a bag. Toss chicken breasts in the dry ingredients. Place seasoned chicken in pan prepared with vegetable cooking spray. Place potatoes and tomatoes over top of chicken. Sprinkle remainder of dry ingredients on the top. Cook uncovered at 400 degrees F for 40 minutes or until done.

Yield: 4 servings

Calories: 369
Exchanges: 4 *Meat*
2 *Bread*
1 *Veg*

Cholesterol: 89 *Mg*
SF: 1 *Gm*
Fat: 4 *Gm*
Sodium: 545 *Mg*
Dietary Fiber: 5 *Gm*

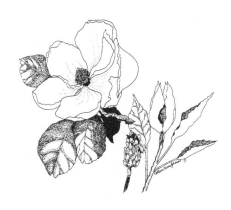

CHICKEN SAUCE PIQUANT

1   pound skinned boneless chicken breast
    dash red pepper
1   teaspoon black pepper
1½ cups chopped bell peppers
3   cups chopped onions
1   cup diced celery
1   teaspoon chili powder
1   can tomato paste
2   cups water
4   ounces light turkey smoked sausage, thinly sliced
    vegetable cooking spray

Cut chicken breasts into strips. Pan fry in non-stick vegetable spray until done. Remove chicken and set aside. Add chopped onion, celery, pepper and cook until tender. Add chili powder, tomato paste, water, seasonings and sausage. Add chicken and cook on low heat for 2 hours.

Yield: 8 servings

Calories: 187
Exchanges: 2 *Meat*
               2 *Vegs*

Cholesterol: 187 *Mg*
SF: 1 *Gm*
Fat: 8 *Gm*
Sodium: 213 *Mg*
Dietary Fiber: 3 *Gm*

SMOTHERED CHICKEN

1	pound chicken breast, skinned
1	cup chopped onions
½	cup diced celery
	olive oil flavored cooking spray
16	ounces fat free chicken broth
3	tablespoons cornstarch
¼	teaspoon black pepper

Spray skillet with cooking spray. Heat on medium high heat. Brown chicken until almost cooked. Add onion, celery and black pepper. Mix cornstarch with chicken broth and pour over chicken and vegetables. Simmer about 25 minutes. Serve over rice.

Yield: 4 (4 ounces of chicken plus ¾ cup vegetables and gravy) servings

Calories: 225
Exchanges: *4   Meat*
                1   Veg

Cholesterol: *87   Mg*
SF: *1   Gm*
Fat: *4   Gm*
Sodium: *253 Mg*
Dietary Fiber: *1   Gm*

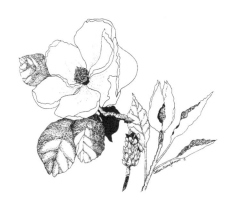

CHICKEN SPAGHETTI

32 ounces skinless, boneless, chicken breasts
1 cup defatted chicken broth
7 ounces raw spaghetti
8 ounces light cheddar cheese
1 cup diced celery
1 cup chopped onion
1 cup chopped bell pepper
1 clove garlic
16 ounces diced canned tomatoes
¼ teaspoon black pepper

Boil chicken. Cut into bite sized pieces Prepare spaghetti according to package directions, omitting any oil. Sauté celery, onion, bell pepper and garlic in cooking spray. Mix spaghetti and chicken with sautéed vegetables. Place in 9" x 13" pan. Add tomato pieces, black pepper and enough chicken broth so that mixture is not dry (about 1 cup). Top with cheese. Bake for 30 minutes at 350 degrees F.

Yield: 12 servings

Calories: 251
Exchanges: *3* *Meat*
               1 *Bread*
               1 *Veg*

Cholesterol: *72 Mg*
SF: *3* *Gm*
Fat: *6* *Gm*
Sodium: *331 Mg*
Dietary Fiber: *2* *Gm*

CHICKEN STEW

1	pound potatoes
2	cups diced celery
12	ounces skinned, boneless chicken breast
1	quart water
1	cup chopped bell pepper
2	ounces tomato paste
½	teaspoon rosemary
½	teaspoon sugar
¼	teaspoon black pepper
	vegetable cooking spray

In a 2½ to 3 quart saucepan, place water, potatoes and 1 cup celery. Bring to a boil. Reduce heat and simmer covered until vegetables are tender, approximately 10 minutes. Set aside. Heat skillet that has been sprayed with cooking spray. Add chicken red pepper and remaining 1 cup of celery. Cook over medium high heat until the chicken is no longer pink. Stir in tomato paste, rosemary, sugar, black pepper and add this mixture back to saucepan. Cook a few minutes longer to thoroughly heat mixture.

Yield: 5 (1 cup) servings

Calories: 196
Exchanges: 2 *Meat*
              1 *Bread*

Cholesterol: 52 *Mg*
SF: 1 *Gm*
Fat: 2 *Gm*
Sodium: 128 *Mg*
Dietary Fiber: 3 *Gm*

MEXICAN CHICKEN STEW

1   **cup cooked chicken**
1   **can (16 ounces) stewed tomatoes**
4   **ounces hot chili peppers**
½   **cup chopped onion**
1   **can (16 ounces) fat free chicken broth**
1   **teaspoon dry bouillon granules**
1   **clove garlic**
¼   **teaspoon cumin**
2   **cups cooked pinto beans**

Combine tomatoes, beans, chili peppers, onion, bouillon granules, garlic powder, cumin and fat free chicken broth. Bring everything to a boil. Reduce heat to low. Cover and simmer approximately 10 minutes. Add chicken and heat to serve.

Yield: 4 (1½ cup) servings

Calories: 259
Exchanges: *2*   *Meat*
               1   *Bread*
               1   *Veg*

Cholesterol: *44 Mg*
SF: *1*   *Gm*
Fat: *3*   *Gm*
Sodium: *501 Mg*
Dietary Fiber: *8*   *Gm*

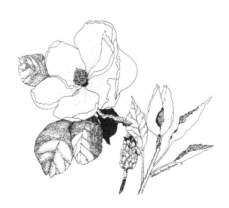

SWEET AND SOUR CHICKEN

     4 tablespoons sweet and sour marinade
     ½ cup water
    1½ teaspoons cornstarch
     8 ounces chicken breast, skinned
     2 cups chopped broccoli
     2 green onions, chopped
     1 cup sliced mushrooms
     3 cups cooked long grain white rice
     3 cups water
        vegetable cooking spray

Refer to index for Sweet and Sour Marinade recipe. Cook 1 cup of rice, which will yield 3 cups of cooked rice, according to package directions omitting oil and salt. Slice chicken into thin small pieces and place in Sweet and Sour Marinade. Add ½ cup water and cornstarch. Set aside. Spray skillet with cooking spray. Heat and add onion and broccoli. Stir fry until onion begins to wilt, but is still crisp. About 2 - 3 minutes. Add chicken and marinade. Cook until chicken turns white and sauce thickens. Serve over ¾ cup rice.

Yield: 4 servings

Calories: 297
Exchanges: *2 Meat*
               1½ Bread
               2 Veg

Cholesterol: *44 Mg*
SF: *1 Gm*
Fat: *2 Gm*
Sodium: *321 Mg*
Dietary Fiber: *2 Gm*

WORKING MOTHER'S CHICKEN

1   pound raw chicken breast, skinned
1   cup long grain white rice
1   cup canned green beans
2   cups water
2   dehydrated chicken cubes
¼   teaspoon black pepper
1   tablespoon dry butter substitute granules

Dissolve chicken broth cubes in hot water. In the bottom of a 2 quart casserole layer in this order: rice, green beans, skinned chicken breast and seasonings. Pour hot broth over casserole. Cover. Place in a 350 degree F oven for approximately 1 hour.

Yield: 6 servings

Calories: 237
Exchanges: *3*   *Meat*
              1   *Bread*
              1   *Veg*

Cholesterol: *58 Mg*
SF: *<1 Gm*
Fat: *3   Gm*
Sodium: *425 Mg*
Dietary Fiber: <1 Gm

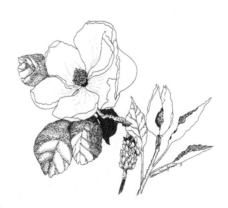

LEMONADE CHICKEN

3   pounds chicken breast, skinned
6   ounces lemonade, canned, frozen concentrate
½   cup lite soy sauce
1   teaspoon Paul Prudhomme's poultry seasoning
¼   teaspoon garlic powder

Combine all ingredients except chicken. Stir well. Set sauce aside. Grill chicken over medium hot coals. After turning once, begin to baste with sauce. Any leftover sauce goes well as a condiment with the meal.

Yield: 12 servings

Calories: 207
Exchanges: 4   Meat
*   ½   Fruit*

Cholesterol: 87   Mg
SF: 1   Gm
Fat: 4   Gm
Sodium: 463 Mg
Dietary Fiber: <1   Gm

BAKED TURKEY BREAST

3   pounds skinned turkey breast
½   teaspoon ground thyme
¼   teaspoon garlic powder
¼   teaspoon black pepper
    vegetable cooking spray

Thaw and wash turkey breast. Remove skin. Spray with cooking spray and rub with seasonings. Place in roasting pan and cover with aluminum foil. Bake in a preheated oven at 325 degrees F for 45 minutes per pound. Serve with cranberry wine sauce.

Yield: 12 (4 ounce) servings

Calories: 154
Exchanges: 5   Meat

Cholesterol: 95   Mg
SF: <1   Gm
Fat: 1   Gm
Sodium: 59   Mg
Dietary Fiber: 0   Gm

LEFT OVER TURKEY AND BROCCOLI CASSEROLE

½ cup chopped onion
½ cup bell chopped pepper
½ cup diced celery
¼ cup liquid Butter Buds
10 ounces (1 package) broccoli spears, frozen
1 cup long grain rice, cooked
1 can (10 ounces) Healthy Request cream of mushroom soup
8 ounces canned water chestnuts
6 ounces fat free cheddar cheese, shredded
¼ teaspoon black pepper
8 ounces turkey breast skinned, cooked and chopped
vegetable cooking spray

Sauté onion, bell pepper and celery in a large skillet that has been treated with cooking spray. Combine remaining ingredients and vegetables. Spoon over broccoli. Bake uncovered at 350 degrees F for 24 - 30 minutes or until thoroughly heated.

Yield: 6 servings

Calories: 168
Exchanges: *1   Meat*
                1   Bread
                1   Veg

Cholesterol: *11   Mg*
SF: *<1   Gm*
Fat: *1   Gm*
Sodium: *515 Mg*
Dietary Fiber: *1   Gm*

TURKEY AND RICE

3	cups wild and white rice mix
10	ounces frozen green peas
1	pound turkey breast, skinned
1	can (4 ounces) water chestnuts
1	ounce sherry wine
4	ounces fat free chicken broth
¼	ounce black pepper
1	tablespoon dry butter substitute granules

Prepare rice mix according to package directions omitting the margarine. Set aside. Cook peas according to package directions. Drain well. Set aside. Combine rice, peas and remaining ingredients. Serve hot with green salad.

Yield: 6 servings

Calories: 222
Exchanges: 2   *Meat*
　　　　　 2   *Bread*
　　　　　 ½   *Veg*

Cholesterol: 10   *Mg*
SF: 1   *Gm*
Fat: 1   *Gm*
Sodium: 563 *Mg*
Dietary Fiber: 2   *Gm*

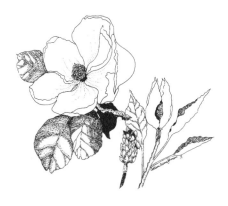

TURKEY ROLLUPS

olive oil flavored cooking spray
½ cup chopped onion
½ cup diced celery
⅓ cup liquid Butter Buds
¼ cup fat free chicken broth
1 teaspoon dried parsley
⅓ cup all purpose flour
¼ teaspoon paprika
1 cup bread crumbs
1½ pounds skinless turkey tenderloins

Pound turkey tenderloin that has been placed between 2 pieces of clear wrap. Divide into eight thin pounded filets. Sauté onion and celery in skillet that has been sprayed with cooking spray. Add bread crumbs, chicken broth, parsley, seasonings, liquid Butter Buds and skim milk. Spoon about ⅓ cut stuffing in the center of each pounded filet of turkey. Roll lengthwise. Tuck edges inside. Secure each roll with a wooden toothpick. Lightly spray baking dish with cooking spray. Dredge turkey rolls in flour and lay in baking dish. Spray each roll with cooking spray and sprinkle with paprika. Excellent served with steamed green vegetables, salad and fat free bread.

Yield: 8 servings

Calories: 159
Exchanges: *3*   *Meat*
             ½   *Bread*

Cholesterol: *71 Mg*
SF: *<1 Gm*
Fat: *1 Gm*
Sodium: *208 Mg*
Dietary Fiber: 1 Gm

QUICK TURKEY ROLLUPS

1	small package stuffing mix
1	cup water
½	cup chopped carrots
½	cup chopped mushrooms
4	ounces liquid Butter Buds
¼	cup flour
8	ounces fat free chicken broth
8	turkey tenderloins
	vegetable cooking spray

Combine the stuffing with hot water, carrots, mushrooms, chicken broth and Butter Buds. Flatten the tenderloins with a tenderizing hammer. Spread each cutlet with 3 tablespoons of mixture. Roll up the cutlets jelly roll style and secure with toothpicks. Roll each cutlet with flour and arrange rolls in casserole sprayed with cooking spray. Place extra stuffing around the rollups. Bake 45 minutes at 350 degrees F.

Yield: 8 servings

Calories: 266
Exchanges: *4*   *Meat*
                 1½ Bread

Cholesterol: *95* *Mg*
SF: *<1* *Gm*
Fat: *2*   *Gm*
Sodium: *662 Mg*
Dietary Fiber: *1*   *Gm*

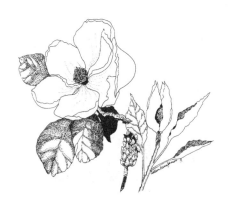

BEEF AND SNOW PEAS

8 ounces thinly sliced top round beef steak
½ cup chopped raw mushrooms
6 ounces of frozen snow pea pods
½ cup chopped onion
1 ounce dry sherry wine
1 tablespoon low salt soy sauce
1⅓ tablespoons cornstarch
1 cup brown rice
vegetable cooking spray

Cook rice according to package directions, omitting any oil or salt. While rice is cooking, slice beef. Marinate sliced beef for 5 minutes in a mixture of sherry, soy sauce and cornstarch. Prepare vegetables. Spray skillet with cooking spray. Heat skillet until very hot. Add beef, cook, about 4-5 minutes, until it loses its pink color. Add vegetables and cook for 1 minute. Add marinade and toss with vegetables for an additional 1 minute. Serve ¼ of meat mixture over ¾ cup of rice.

Yield: 4 servings

Calories: 296
Exchanges: 2   *Meat*
                2   *Bread*
                1   *Veg*

Cholesterol: 25   *Mg*
SF: 1   *Gm*
Fat: 3   *Gm*
Sodium: 565   *Mg*
Dietary Fiber: 3   *Gm*

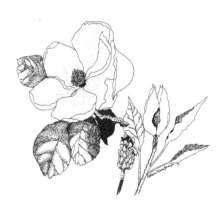

BEEF POT PIE

2 cups cubed potatoes
1 cup sliced carrots
1 cup chopped onion
1 clove garlic
½ teaspoon salt
¼ teaspoon black pepper
¼ teaspoon thyme
1 bay leaf
4 cups water
6 small whole onions
1 cup diced celery
¼ cup skim milk
2 tablespoons cornstarch
2 pounds Healthy Choice ground beef
1 can Pillsbury light biscuits
  vegetable cooking spray

Brown meat in a large Dutch oven that has been sprayed with cooking spray. Add onion, garlic, salt, pepper, thyme, bay leaf and water. Cover, reduce heat and simmer for 30 minutes. Add potatoes, carrots, small onions and celery. Cover and cook over low heat for 15 minutes. Remove a small amount of broth and put in a cup. Add ¼ cup skim milk and 3 tablespoons cornstarch. Stir to dissolve the cornstarch. Pour back into the pot to thicken the gravy. Open a can of light biscuits and place on top. Place in an a 400 degree F oven. Cover and cook for an additional 12 - 15 minutes, until the biscuits are done.

Yield: 10 servings

Calories: 186
Exchanges: 2 *Meat*
              1 *Bread*
              1 *Veg*

Cholesterol: 28 *Mg*
SF: 1 *Gm*
Fat: 4 *Gm*
Sodium: 335 *Mg*
Dietary Fiber: 1 *Gm*

BEEF POTLUCK CASSEROLE

1 pound Healthy Choice ground beef
1 cup chopped onions
½ cup chopped bell pepper
6 ounces raw pasta noodles
1 can Campbell's Healthy Request cream of mushroom
   soup
8 ounces frozen mixed vegetables
¼ cup low-fat cheddar cheese, shredded
   vegetable cooking spray

Brown meat, onions and bell peppers in non-stick vegetable spray. Cook noodles without fat and drain. Cook vegetables until tender. Combine meat, noodles, soup and mixed vegetables. Pour into baking dish. Top with ¼ cup low fat cheddar cheese. Bake at 350 degrees F until bubbly and cheese melts.

Yield: 8 servings

Calories: 197
Exchanges: *1*   *Meat*
            1   *Bread*
            1   *Veg*

Cholesterol: *53 Mg*
SF: *1   Gm*
Fat: *4   Gm*
Sodium: *275 Mg*
Dietary Fiber: 1   Gm

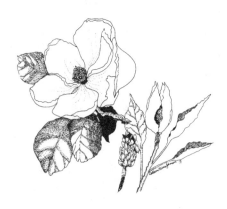

HOMESTYLE CHILI

2 pounds of Healthy Choice ground beef
2 cups chopped onions
2 cloves garlic
1 teaspoon salt
¼ teaspoon black pepper
3 cups water
¼ teaspoon red pepper
1 tablespoon all purpose flour
¼ cup chili powder
1 6 ounce can tomato paste
1 tablespoon cumin
2 small cans pinto beans, drained
   vegetable cooking spray

Lean venison may be substituted for Healthy Choice ground beef, giving approximately the same fat grams per serving.

Brown meat, onions, and garlic in vegetable cooking spray. Add salt, pepper, cumin, red pepper and sprinkle flour over mixture in pan. Mix together boiling water and chili powder. Add to meat. Add drained beans to mixture. Cook slowly 1 hour. Add tomato paste. Cook 30 minutes longer.

Yield: 10 (1 cup) servings

Calories: 197
Exchanges: *2   Meat*
              1   Bread
              1   Veg

Cholesterol: *45 Mg*
SF: *1   Gm*
Fat: *4   Gm*
Sodium: *784 Mg*
Dietary Fiber: *2   Gm*

GRILLED HAMBURGER WITH CHEESE

1 **pound Healthy Choice ground beef**
5 **hamburger buns**
¼ **cup egg substitute**
¼ **teaspoon garlic powder**
¼ **teaspoon salt**
2 **ounces fat free American cheese**
2 **tablespoons dehydrated onion flakes**

Soak 1 bun in ¼ cup water. Drain water and crumble 1 bun into meat. Add egg substitute, onion, seasonings and garlic powder. Divide meat in to 4 meatballs. Stuff each meatball with cheese. Grill 4 minutes on each side. Use fat free mayonnaise, mustard, lettuce and tomato.

Yield: 4 servings

Calories: 267
Exchanges: *3 Meat*
            2 Bread

Cholesterol: *56 Mg*
SF: *1 Gm*
Fat: *6 Gm*
Sodium: *674 Mg*
Dietary Fiber: *1 Gm*

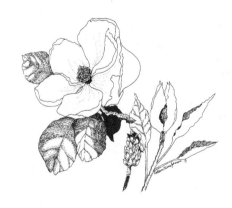

HAMBURGER PIE

1½ pounds Healthy Choice hamburger
1   can corn
¼   cup chopped bell pepper
1   can chopped whole tomatoes
1⅓ cups chopped onions
¼   teaspoon salt
1   package Jiffy cornbread mix
¼   cup egg substitute
⅓   cup skim milk
    vegetable cooking spray

Sauté beef, bell pepper, and onion. Drain. Add drained corn and chopped to-matoes to this mixture. Place in a casserole dish prepared with cooking spray. Mix cornbread mix with egg substitute and skim milk in a medium bowl until well blended. Pour on top of meat ingredients in casserole. Bake at 350 de-grees F for 25 to 30 minutes.

Yield: 9 servings

Calories: 186
Exchanges: 2½ *Meat*
                 1 *Bread*
                 1 *Veg*

Cholesterol: 38 *Mg*
SF: 1 *Gm*
Fat: 5 *Gm*
Sodium: 532 *Mg*
Dietary Fiber: 1 *Gm*

HAMBURGER STROGANOFF

1 pound Healthy Choice ground beef
½ cup chopped onions
1 clove garlic
   butter flavored cooking spray
¼ cup dry butter substitute
2 tablespoons all purpose flour
¼ teaspoon black pepper
8 ounces canned mushrooms
6 ounces Campbell's Healthy Request cream of
   mushroom soup
8 ounces fat free sour cream
1 tablespoon parsley

Sauté onion and garlic in vegetable spray. Add meat and brown. Add flour, seasonings, butter substitute and mushrooms. Cook for 5 minutes. Add soup and simmer uncovered for 10 minutes. Before serving, stir in fat free sour cream. Heat thoroughly and garnish with parsley. Serve over noodles or rice.

Yield: 6 servings

Calories: 147
Exchanges: *1 Meat*
             ½ Bread
             1 Milk

Cholesterol: *38 Mg*
SF: *1 Gm*
Fat: *3 Gm*
Sodium: *522 Mg*
Dietary Fiber: *1 Gm*

EASY LASAGNE

1 pound Healthy Choice ground beef
16 ounces hot and spicy vegetable juice
16 ounces fat free cottage cheese
12 ounces fat free shredded Mozzarella cheese
½ cup egg substitute (or 2 egg whites may be substituted)
¼ teaspoon black pepper
8 ounces lasagne noodles
¼ cup fat free Parmesan cheese
28 ounces light spaghetti sauce
vegetable cooking spray

Spray skillet with cooking spray. Brown ground beef. Add sauce and juice to meat. Set aside. Mix the cottage cheese and the shredded Mozzarella, egg substitute and seasonings. Set aside. Pour 1 cup sauce into the bottom of a 9" x 12" pan. Place 3 uncooked noodles on top of the sauce. (The noodles will expand and absorb the liquid as they cook). Add ½ of the cheese filling. Repeat sauce, noodles and filling. Top with layer of noodles and remaining sauce. Cover with aluminum foil and bake at 350 degrees F for 1 hour. Remove foil and sprinkle with ¼ cup fat free Parmesan cheese and bake an additional 10 minutes. Allow to stand 10 minutes before slicing.

Yield: 9 servings

Calories: 226
Exchanges: *3* *Meat*
               1 *Bread*
               1 *Veg*

Cholesterol: *36 Mg*
SF: *<1 Gm*
Fat: *2 Gm*
Sodium: *945 Mg*
Dietary Fiber: *2 Gm*

MEXICAN LASAGNA

1½ pounds Healthy Choice ground beef
1 16 ounce can stewed diced tomatoes
1½ teaspoons ground cumin
1 teaspoon chili powder
¼ teaspoon red pepper
1 teaspoon black pepper
¼ teaspoon garlic powder
¼ teaspoon salt
10 frozen tortillas (thawed)
2 cups fat free cottage cheese
4 ounces low fat Monterey Jack cheese
¼ cup egg substitute
2 cups shredded lettuce
½ cup diced tomato
3 chopped green onions

Brown meat, drain if necessary. Add the next 7 ingredients. Heat thoroughly. Cover bottom and sides of 13" x 9" pan with tortillas. Pour beef mixture over tortillas. Place a layer of tortillas over meat mixture. Combine cottage cheese, Monterey Jack cheese with egg substitute. Pour over tortillas. Bake at 350 degrees F for 30 minutes. Remove and garnish with lettuce, diced tomatoes and green onions.

Yield: 9 servings

Calories: 243
Exchanges: *3*   *Meat*
             1   *Bread*
             ½   *Veg*

Cholesterol: *45 Mg*
SF: *1*   *Gm*
Fat: *5*   *Gm*
Sodium: *724 Mg*
Dietary Fiber: *2*   *Gm*

MEATBALLS AND SPAGHETTI

1 pound Healthy Choice ground beef
2 egg whites
½ cup bread crumbs
2 tablespoons parsley
⅛ teaspoon black pepper
28 ounces non-fat spaghetti sauce
12 ounces pasta
   vegetable cooking spray

In a large bowl, combine ground beef, eggs whites, bread crumbs, parsley and pepper. Shape into 8 meat balls, approximately 1½" in diameter (you may desire to make meatballs smaller) and place on a baking sheet that has been sprayed with cooking spray. Bake meatballs about 30 minutes at 350 degrees F or until well browned. Transfer cooked meatballs to a large saucepan. Add non-fat spaghetti sauce, cover and simmer for 30 minutes. Serve sauce and meatballs over hot cooked spaghetti. Cook according to package directions, eliminating fat.

Yield: 8 servings

Calories: 165
Exchanges: *1½ Meat*
           1 Bread
           ½ Veg

Cholesterol: *28 Mg*
SF: *<1 Gm*
Fat: *3 Gm*
Sodium: *534 Mg*
Dietary Fiber: *3 Gm*

MEATLOAF

1½   pounds of Healthy Choice ground beef
¾   cup raw oatmeal
1   cup chopped onions
½   cup chopped bell pepper
8   ounces canned tomato sauce
8   ounces tomato catsup
¼   cup egg substitute
     dash black pepper
     vegetable cooking spray

Mix beef, oatmeal, onion, bell pepper, 4 ounces catsup and 4 ounces tomato sauce, egg substitute and pepper. Shape into a loaf. Place in loaf pan that has been prepared with vegetable cooking spray. Bake at 350 degrees F for 45 - 50 minutes. Pour remaining sauce and catsup over meatloaf and bake another 20 minutes.

Yield: 8 servings

Calories: 182
Exchanges: 2   *Meat*
                 ½   *Bread*
                 ½   *Veg*

Cholesterol: 42 *Mg*
SF: 1   *Gm*
Fat: 4   *Gm*
Sodium: 716 *Mg*
Dietary Fiber: 2   *Gm*

PIGS IN A BLANKET

8 Healthy Choice wieners
8 Ballard light biscuits
   vegetable cooking spray

Open can of light biscuits. Roll each individual biscuit out using a rolling pin or plastic glass. Lay a wiener on one end of a biscuit. Roll up until dough goes completely around the wiener. Repeat until you have rolled each wiener with a biscuit. Place on a cookie sheet that has been sprayed with vegetable cooking spray. Bake at 400 degrees F for approximately 8 minutes or until bread is lightly browned.

Yield: 8 servings

Calories: 101
Exchanges: 1   Meat
*   1   Bread*

Cholesterol: 15 Mg
SF: 1   Gm
Fat: 2   Gm
Sodium: 630 Mg
Dietary Fiber: 0   Gm

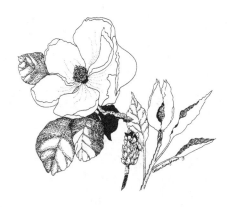

PIZZA CASSEROLE

1 pound Healthy Choice ground beef
1 jar (14 ounces) pizza sauce
8 ounces fat free Mozzarella cheese
6 ounces low fat biscuit mix
1½ cups skim milk
½ cup egg substitute

Cook ground beef in a skillet over medium heat until brown. Stir to crumble. Drain. Spoon beef into an 8" square baking pan. Top with pizza sauce and cheese. Combine biscuit mix, milk and egg substitute. Beat until smooth. Pour mixture over casserole. Cover evenly. Bake at 400 degrees F for 30 - 35 minutes.

Yield: 6 servings

Calories: 314
Exchanges: *4* *Meat*
    1½ *Bread*
    1 *Veg*

Cholesterol: *45* *Mg*
SF: *1* *Gm*
Fat: *4* *Gm*
Sodium: *999* *Mg*
Dietary Fiber: *0* *Gm*

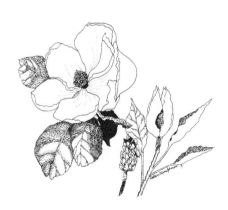

DEEP DISH PIZZA

6 ounces Healthy Choice ground beef
1 cup fat free spaghetti sauce
  olive oil flavored cooking spray
1 cup chopped onions
½ cup chopped bell pepper
1½ teaspoons garlic powder
2 tablespoons cornmeal
2 (11 ounce) packages refrigerated French bread dough
3 ounces fat free Mozzarella cheese
2 ounces Romano cheese

Cook ground beef, onion and bell pepper over medium-high heat until browned, stirring to crumble. Drain and set aside. Coat 2 (9") cake pans with cooking spray and sprinkle each with 1 teaspoon of cornmeal. Unroll bread dough, folding each corner in toward the center of pan to form a round shape. Spread ½ cup sauce over each crust. Top each with ½ of meat mixture. Sprinkle ¼ cup Mozzarella cheese and 2 tablespoons of Romano cheese on each crust. Bake at 475 degrees F for 12 minutes. Let stand 5 minutes. Cut each pizza into 4 wedges.

Yield: 8 servings

Calories 173
Exchanges: 1 *Meat*
              1 *Bread*
              ½ *Veg*
              ½ *Fat*

Cholesterol: 21 *Mg*
SF: 2 *Gm*
Fat: 5 *Gm*
Sodium   370 *Mg*
Dietary Fiber: 2 *Gm*

PIZZA ROLL

1   loaf frozen bread dough
1   cup chopped onions
¼   cup chopped bell pepper
1   pound Healthy Choice ground beef
8   ounces shredded fat free cheddar cheese
    butter flavored vegetable spray
4   tablespoons fat free spaghetti sauce
½   cup fresh mushrooms, sliced

Thaw dough at room temperature for approximately 1½ hours or overnight in the refrigerator. Sauté onion, bell pepper and mushrooms in cooking spray until tender. Set aside. Brown meat and drain. Set aside. Roll out bread dough to ¼" thickness. Mix meat with vegetable mixture and sauce. Spread this mixture over dough. Follow with cheese. Roll up "jelly roll" fashion. Spray with cooking spray and bake at 350 degrees F for 20 to 30 minutes or until brown. Let stand 10 minutes before slicing.

Yield: 8 servings

Calories: 181
Exchanges: *½   Meat*
                1   Bread
                1   Fat
                1   Veg

Cholesterol: 28 Mg
SF: <1 Gm
Fat: 4   Gm
Sodium: 576 Mg
Dietary Fiber: 2   Gm

SOUTH OF THE BORDER PIZZA

½   **pound Healthy Choice ground beef**
1   **package low salt taco seasoning**
6   **ounces tomato paste**
1   **cup water**
1   **box (16 ounces) hot roll mix**
4   **ounces light cheddar cheese**
    vegetable cooking spray

Brown ½ pound of Healthy Choice ground beef in cooking spray. Stir in taco seasoning, tomato paste and water. Prepare pizza dough as directed on the hot roll mix. Push dough into a greased 9" x 13" pan. Cover. Let stand 15 minutes. Spread meat mixture over dough. Top with cheese. Bake in 275 degree F oven for 20 minutes.

Yield: 9 servings

Calories: 306
Exchanges: *1½ Meat*
          2   Bread
          ½   Veg

Cholesterol: *41 Mg*
SF: *1   Gm*
Fat: *7   Gm*
Sodium: *820 Mg*
Dietary Fiber: *1   Gm*

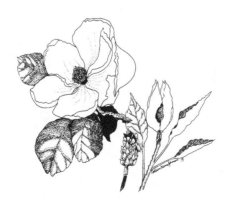

SUNDAY ROAST

2	pounds beef eye of round
⅛	teaspoon salt
⅛	teaspoon black pepper
8 - 10	new potatoes
3	ribs of celery, cut in large pieces
3	cups peeled and cubed carrots
1	cup brewed coffee
2	tablespoons cornstarch

Salt and pepper roast and place in a Dutch oven. Pour 1 cup of liquid coffee over roast. Place potatoes, carrots, and celery on sides of roast. Cover and cook for 2 hours or until meat is tender/done. Remove roast and vegetables. Place broth in freezer for several minutes until fat rises to top. Skim off fat. Thicken broth with cornstarch. Add meat back to gravy and heat thoroughly.

Yield: 8 (4 ounces roast with 1 cup vegetables) servings

Calories: 280
Exchanges: *4*   *Meat*
              1   *Bread*
              2   *Vegs*

Cholesterol: *79 Mg*
SF: *2*   *Gm*
Fat: *6*   *Gm*
Sodium: *155 Mg*
Dietary Fiber: *2*   *Gm*

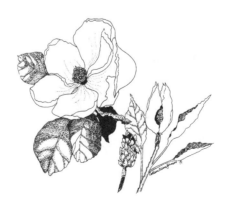

MAMA B'S SPAGHETTI

2 pounds Healthy choice ground beef
1 cup chopped onions
1 tablespoon dehydrated onion flakes
1 teaspoon ground oregano
¼ teaspoon ground thyme
1 tablespoon chili powder
1 tablespoon sugar
1 tablespoon Mrs. Dash seasoning
½ cup water
1 can (16 ounces) tomato sauce
1 can (16 ounces) whole tomatoes
1 package (16 ounces) spaghetti
vegetable cooking spray

Brown meat in skillet that has been sprayed with cooking spray. Drain if necessary. Add onion. Cook until transparent, about 10 minutes. Add onion flakes, oregano, thyme, Mrs. Dash, chili powder and water. Simmer 45 minutes. Add sugar. Cook spaghetti according to package directions without adding oil.

Yield: 16 (1 ounce spaghetti and ¾ cup sauce) servings

Calories: 194
Exchanges: *2* *Meat*
          1½ Bread
          1 *Veg*

Cholesterol: *28 Mg*
SF: *1* *Gm*
Fat: *3* *Gm*
Sodium: *394 Mg*
Dietary Fiber: *1* *Gm*

STEAK AND GRAVY

2   **pounds top round steak (tenderized)**
1½ **cups water**
½   **cup brewed coffee**
2   **beef bouillon cubes**
2   **cups chopped onions**
3   **tablespoons cornstarch**
     vegetable cooking spray

Tenderize round steak by using a tenderizing hammer or you may purchase meat that has already been tenderized at the market. Cut meat into 4 ounce servings or strips. Dissolve bouillon cubes in water. Add coffee and cornstarch. Set aside. Spray skillet with vegetable cooking spray. In a hot skillet, brown meat. The last few minutes before meat is completely done, add onions. Cook until wilted or slightly browned, depending upon your personal preference. Add broth mixture. Bring to a boil. Lower heat to a simmer. Cover and cook for about 30 minutes. Serve over rice with a green vegetable.

Yield: 4 servings

Calories: 204
Exchanges: *4   Meat*
                1   Veg

Cholesterol: *71 Mg*
SF: *2   Gm*
Fat: *5   Gm*
Sodium: *489 Mg*
Dietary Fiber: *<1 Gm*

STEAK ON A STICK

¼ cup wine
1 tablespoon lite soy sauce
1½ teaspoons balsamic vinegar
1½ teaspoons tomato catsup
1½ teaspoons honey
⅛ teaspoon garlic powder
1 pound sirloin steak

Combine first 6 ingredients in a large hallow dish. Add steak that has been cut into 1" cubes. Cover and marinate for 2 hours in refrigerator. Turn occasionally. Drain steak. Reserve marinade. Thread steak on 7" skewers. (If you do not have skewers, they may be found at the grocery store or gourmet kitchen shop). Grill 5 minutes on each side, basting with marinade, over medium coals or until desired doneness.

Yield: 5 (3 ounce) servings

Calories: 216
Exchanges: 3   Meat

Cholesterol: 81   Mg
SF: 3   Gm
Fat: 7   Gm
Sodium: 192 Mg
Dietary Fiber: 0   Gm

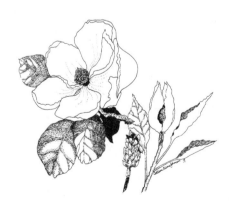

TAMALE PIE

1½ cups cold water
1½ cups cornmeal
 1 teaspoon salt
 2 cups boiling water
 ½ cup chopped onion
 2 tablespoons all purpose flour
16 ounce can sliced stewed tomatoes
 8 ounce can tomato sauce
1½ cups cooked frozen kernels of corn
 2 pounds Healthy Choice ground beef
 3 tablespoons chili powder
   vegetable cooking spray

Combine cold water and cornmeal. Add ½ teaspoon salt to boiling water. Add cornmeal mixture, stirring constantly, bring back to boil. Partially cover pan. Turn heat down and cook for 7 minutes, stirring often. Spray bottom and sides of a 2 quart casserole with non-stick cooking spray. Line the bottom and sides with cornmeal mush. Set aside. Brown beef and onion in skilled sprayed with cooking spray. Stir in flour, remaining salt and chili powder. Add tomatoes, tomato sauce and corn. Pour into a casserole lined with cornmeal mush.

Yield: 6 servings

Calories: 318
Exchanges: 2 *Meat*
          2 *Bread*
          2 *Veg*

Cholesterol: 37 *Mg*
SF: 1 *Gm*
Fat: 4 *Gm*
Sodium: 768 *Mg*
Dietary Fiber: 5 *Gm*

SMOKED HAM AND CABBAGE

	vegetable cooking spray
5	cups raw cabbage, sliced
1	cup chopped onions
1	cup diced carrots
1	can kidney beans
1	can stewed tomatoes
1	tablespoon vinegar
1½	ounces Parmesan cheese
2	tablespoons all purpose flour
	dash of black pepper
12	ounces Healthy Choice baked ham

Heat oven to 350 degrees F. Prepare Dutch oven with non-stick spray. Place over medium-high heat. Add cabbage, onion and carrots and sauté for 5 minutes. Stir in beans, tomatoes and vinegar. Sprinkle cheese, flour and pepper over cabbage mixture. Stir. Spoon into 2 quart casserole that has been sprayed with non-stick cooking spray. Cut ham in bite sized pieces. Arrange on top of cabbage mixture and cover. Bake 40 minutes or until hot.

Yield: 6 servings

Calories: 281
Exchanges: 2 *Meat*
1 *Bread*
2 *Veg*

Cholesterol:: 33 *Mg*
SF: 1 *Gm*
Fat: 4 *Gm*
Sodium: 853 *Mg*
Dietary Fiber: 8 *Gm*

SOUTHERN PRALINE HAM

3 **pounds Healthy Choice honey ham**
16 **ounces jar of apricot or plum jam or preserves**
½ **cup packed brown sugar**

Follow package directions for heating precooked ham. Combine preserves
with brown sugar. Heat in microwave for 1 minute, stir. Continue heating
until warm and liquid. Spread over ham for last hour of baking.

Yield: 16 (3 ounce) servings

Calories: 188
Exchanges: *2*   *Meat*
                 ½   *Bread*

Cholesterol: *35 Mg*
SF: *1   Gm*
Fat: *3   Gm*
Sodium: *772 Mg*
Dietary Fiber: *1   Gm*

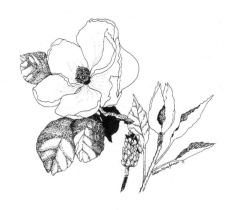

PORK CHOPS AND VEGETABLES

1½   pounds pork loin chop
½   cup of chopped green peppers
2   tablespoons flour
1   can Healthy Request cream of chicken soup
2   tablespoons Worcestershire sauce
1   teaspoon garlic powder
16   ounces tomato puree
     vegetable cooking spray

In a large skillet sprayed with non-stick cooking spray, brown pork chops on both sides. Remove and set aside. Add green peppers to skillet and sauté for 2 minutes. Stir in flour, onion soup, Worcestershire sauce and garlic powder. Bring to a boil. Add chops back to skillet. Cover and simmer until tender, about 1 hour. Stir in tomatoes. Cook an additional 5 minutes. Serve with rice and a green salad.

Yield: 6 servings

Calories: 271
Exchanges: 4   *Meat*
              ½   *Bread*
              2   *Veg*

Cholesterol: 67 *Mg*
SF: 3   *Gm*
Fat: 10 *Gm*
Sodium: 496 *Mg*
Dietary Fiber: 2   *Gm*

STUFFED ROAST PORK TENDERLOIN

1   pound lean pork tenderloin
1   tablespoon all purpose flour
3   tablespoons cornstarch
½   cup defatted chicken broth
     vegetable cooking spray
     cooking bag
     kitchen string

STUFFING INGREDIENTS:

1   cup chopped onion
½   cup raw celery
1   clove of garlic
1   bay leaf crumbled
     dash of black pepper
1   cup cooked wild rice

Trim all visible fat from pork. Split meat in half lengthwise, stopping about ½" from the edge. Open the split and flatten the meat.

Sauté onions, garlic, celery and bay leaf in vegetable cooking spray until tender. Add 1 cup cooked wild rice and mix. Spread stuffing mixture inside the split meat. Fold meat back over itself. Tie at 1" spaces with kitchen string. Place flour in cooking and shake to coat the interior of the bag. Add the meat and broth and tie the bag shut. Place the bag in a shallow baking pan. Bake at 350 degrees F until meat reaches an internal temperature of 165 degrees F, about an hour.

GRAVY:

Chill broth in freezer for about 10 minutes. Skim off fat. Thicken with cornstarch over low heat for several minutes.

Yield: 4 servings (4 ounces each)

Calories: 261
Exchanges: *4*   *Meat*
              ½   *Bread*
              ½   *Veg*

Cholesterol: *105 Mg*
SF: *2*   *Gm*
Fat: *6*   *Gm*
Sodium: *103 Mg*
Dietary Fiber: *2*   *Gm*

SWEET AND SOUR PORK

- 1½   **pounds center cut pork loin**
- 13½   **ounces water packed pineapple bits**
- ¼   **cup distilled vinegar**
-      **dash of salt**
- ¼   **teaspoon garlic powder**
- 2   **tablespoons sugar**
- 1   **cup rice**
- ½   **chopped cup green peppers**
-      **vegetable cooking spray**

Spray skillet with cooking spray. Brown meat over medium heat. Drain pineapple tidbits. Mix juice with enough water to make 2½ cups. Add to juice and water mixture, vinegar, salt and sugar. Pour into skillet with pork and bring to a boil. Reduce heat to low and simmer covered for 20 minutes. Remove cover, stir in rice. Cover and continue cooking for 25 minutes or longer, until rice is tender and the liquid has been absorbed. Add pineapple tidbits and green pepper. Heat thoroughly.

Yield: 6 servings

Calories: 322
Exchanges: 4   *Meat*
             1   *Bread*
             1   *Fruit*

Cholesterol: 66 *Mg*
SF: 2   *Gm*
Fat: 7   *Gm*
Sodium   251 *Mg*
Dietary Fiber: 1   *Gm*

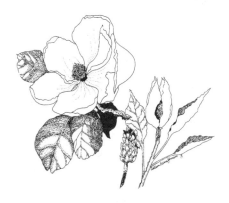

QUAIL ON BROWN RICE

8   (approximately 1 pound) quail breasts
1   cup chopped onion
1   cup diced celery
½   cup chopped bell pepper
2   tablespoons Worcestershire
1   tablespoon garlic powder
½   teaspoon salt
¼   teaspoon red pepper
1   can Healthy Request cream of mushroom soup
½   cup water
2   cups cooked brown rice
2   slices chopped Canadian bacon
     vegetable cooking spray

Sauté Canadian bacon in skillet until crisp. Remove, drain on paper towels. Sauté onion, bell pepper, and celery in vegetable spray. Add quail and Canadian bacon to vegetable mixture. Stir in Worcestershire sauce, garlic, salt, pepper , soup and water. Mix well. Bring to boil. Reduce heat and simmer for 30 minutes.

Yield: 4 servings (2 quail breast and 1 cup rice mixture)

Calories: 327
Exchanges: *4   Meat*
                1½ bread
                1   Veg

Cholesterol: *8   Mg*
SF: *2   Gm*
Fat: *6   Gm*
Sodium: *770 Mg*
Dietary Fiber: *4   Gm*

HUNTER'S VENISON ROAST

3   pounds lean venison roast
3   cups sliced carrots
6   cups onions, quartered
6   cups potatoes, quartered
1   can Healthy Request cream of mushroom soup
1   cup all purpose flour
2   tablespoons Worcestershire sauce
1   teaspoon salt
1   tablespoon black pepper
1   teaspoon garlic powder
3   cups water

Place venison, carrots, onions, potatoes, soup, flour, Worcestershire sauce, salt, garlic and pepper in browning bag. Add water. Close bag and place in roasting pan. Bake at 350 degrees F for 3 hours.

Yield: 10 servings

Calories: 423
Exchanges: *5*   *Meat*
                 2   *bread*
                 1   *Veg*

Cholesterol: *112 Mg*
SF: *1   Gm*
Fat: *4   Gm*
Sodium: *446 Mg*
Dietary Fiber: *6   Gm*

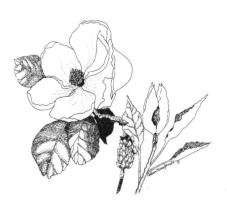

TEX MEX VENISON STEW

1½ **pounds ground lean venison**
¼ **cup all purpose flour**
    vegetable cooking spray
1 **cup chopped onions**
1 **clove garlic**
1 **can (4 ounces) hot chili peppers**
1 **teaspoon black pepper**
8 **ounces red wine**
1 **can (15 ounces) canned tomato sauce**
1 **can fat free beef broth**

Dredge meat in flour. Cook in hot skillet that has been sprayed with cooking spray. Add remaining ingredients. Stir and cover. Reduce heat and simmer 2½ hours. Stir occasionally. Great served with baked tortilla chips, cornbread or rice.

Yield: 16 (1 cup) servings

Calories: 257
Exchanges: *2* *Meat*
               1 *Veg*

Cholesterol: *93* *Mg*
SF: *1* *Gm*
Fat: *2* *Gm*
Sodium: *736 Mg*
Dietary Fiber: *2* *Gm*

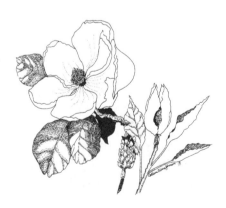

RED BEANS AND RICE

- **4** ounces cubed lean ham
- **8** cups water
- **5** cloves garlic
- **¼** teaspoon Louisiana hot sauce
- **2** bay leaves
- **¼** teaspoon salt
- **1** pound red kidney beans, dry, uncooked
- **1** cup diced celery
- **1** cup chopped onion
  vegetable cooking spray
- **½** pound light smoked sausage
- **1** teaspoon Worcestershire sauce
- **¼** teaspoon black pepper
- **¼** cup chopped fresh parsley
- **6** cups cooked rice

Wash and soak beans. Drain. In a large pot, place ham, water, garlic, hot sauce, Worcestershire sauce and beans. Cook uncovered over low heat. In another pan, sauté celery, onions and garlic in cooking spray. Add to bean mixture. Add sausage, sliced thin and remaining seasonings to bean mixture. Cook 2½ hours. Remove bay leaves and serve over hot rice prepared with added fat or salt.

Yield: 12 (⅔ cup red beans over ½ cup rice) servings

Calories: 201
Exchanges: *1   Meat*
                2   Bread
Cholesterol: *7   Mg*
SF: *<1 Gm*
Fat: *4   Gm*
Sodium: *218 Mg*
Dietary Fiber: *2   Gm*

VEGETABLE LASAGNE

28	ounces fat free spaghetti sauce
2	cups raw, sliced zucchini squash
2	cups raw sliced yellow squash
½	cup shredded carrot
6	lasagna noodles
12	ounces fat free ricotta cheese
1⅓	ounces fat free Parmesan cheese
½	teaspoons ground oregano
8	ounces low fat Mozzarella cheese

Heat oven to 350 degrees F. Mix spaghetti sauce and vegetables. Spread 1½ cups sauce mixture in a baking dish (13" x 9" x 2"). Top with 3 uncooked noodles. Mix Ricotta and Parmesan cheese and oregano. Spread over noodles in dish. Add 1½ cups sauce mixture and spread evenly. Top with remaining noodles and sauce. Sprinkle top with Mozzarella cheese. Bake uncovered for 45 minutes. Let stand 15 minutes before cutting.

Yield: 12 servings

Calories: 174
Exchanges: *1*   *Meat*
                1   *Bread*
                1   *Veg*
Cholesterol: *22 Mg*
SF: *2*   *Gm*
Fat: *3*   *Gm*
Sodium: *487 Mg*
Dietary Fiber: *2*   *Gm*

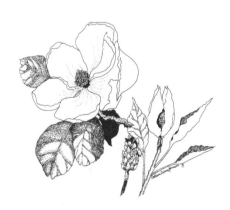

VEGETABLES AND STARCHES

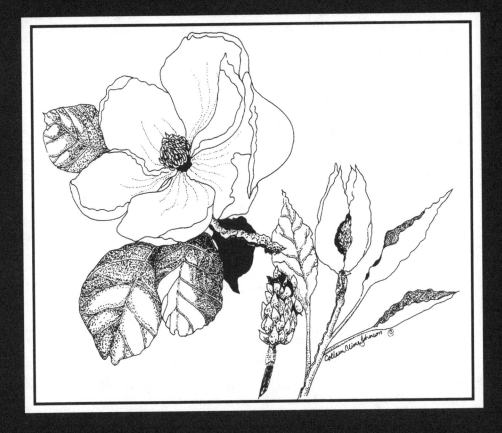

Colleen Cline Johnson ©

BROILED FRESH ASPARAGUS

  vegetable cooking spray
1 pound fresh asparagus
¼ teaspoon garlic salt
2 tablespoons Parmesan cheese, grated

Preheat broiler in oven to 400 degrees F. Spray jelly roll pan with olive oil flavored non-stick cooking spray. Lay asparagus on pan. Spray lightly with cooking spray. Sprinkle with garlic salt and Parmesan cheese. Broil about 3 minutes. Watch closely. Do not allow vegetables to scorch. This an excellent dish to serve with grilled fish or chicken and wild rice.

Yield: 6 servings

Calories: 27
Exchanges: *1   Veg*

Cholesterol: *2   Mg*
SF: *<1   Gm*
Fat: *1   Gm*
Sodium: *131 Mg*
Dietary Fiber: *1   Gm*

GREEN BEANS DIJON

1 tablespoon balsamic vinegar
¼ teaspoon Dijon mustard
1 clove garlic
½ teaspoon ground oregano
½ teaspoon black pepper
1 pound frozen green beans

Steam beans for 3 to 4 minutes. While beans are steaming, mix all other ingredients in a bowl. Add beans and toss to coat with sauce.

Yield: 4 servings

Calories: 36
Exchanges: *2   Veg*

Cholesterol: *8   Mg*
SF: *0   Gm*
Fat: *<1   Gm*
Sodium: *46   Mg*
Dietary Fiber: *0   Gm*

LIGHT GREEN BEANS WITH SOUR CREAM

¼ cup onion, chopped
4 tablespoons butter substitute granules
¼ cup water
2 tablespoons all purpose flour
1 teaspoon sugar
2 ounces pimientos
8 ounces fat free sour cream
1 ounce light ranch style dressing
8 ounces light Swiss cheese
4 cups can green beans, drained

Preheat oven to 350 degrees F. Mix butter substitute, water, flour, salt, sugar, onion and pimientos. Stir until well mixed. Add the sour cream and salad dressing. Cook until sauce is thick. Fold in beans and Swiss cheese. Transfer to a 2 quart casserole dish and bake 20 minutes.

Yield: 8 servings

Calories: 124
Exchanges: *1   Meat*
               1   Veg

Cholesterol: *15 Gm*
SF: *2   Gm*
Fat: *3   Gm*
Sodium: *867 Mg*
Dietary Fiber: *1   Gm*

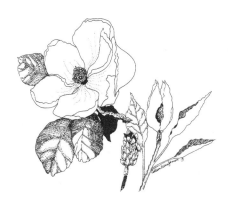

SUNDAY GREEN BEANS

20 ounces frozen green beans
    olive oil flavored cooking spray
½ cup chopped onion
2 tablespoons all purpose flour
1 tablespoon dry butter substitute
   dash black pepper
8 ounces fat free sour cream
2 ounces light cheddar cheese

Steam beans until thawed, but still crisp (about 3 minutes). Drain. Cook onions in saucepan that has been sprayed with cooking spray. Mix sour cream, flour and black pepper. Add sour cream mixture to onions. Heat thoroughly. Do not boil. Add beans and pour into a 2 quart casserole. Top with cheese. Bake at 350 degrees F for 15 minutes or until cheese melts.

Yield: 8 servings

Calories: 63
Exchanges: *1*   *Veg*

Cholesterol: *4*   *Mg*
SF: *1*   *Gm*
Fat: *1*   *Gm*
Sodium: *143 Mg*
Dietary Fiber: *1*   *Gm*

FRESH SNAP BEANS AND HERBS

1 **pound fresh snap beans**
1 **tablespoon butter substitute granules**
½ **teaspoon dried rosemary**
½ **teaspoon dried basil**

If fresh herbs are used, use 2 teaspoons of each.

You can buy fresh snap beans at the Farmer's Market or in the grocery store. If you cannot find fresh ones in your area, look for young tender whole beans at the grocer's. Steam beans until almost tender, about 6 minutes in a steamer. Drain. Stir in the remain ingredients. Place vegetables in a microwave safe casserole dish. Set aside. When meal is ready to serve, place vegetables in the microwave just to warm (about 1 minute).

Yield: 4 servings

Calories: 38
Exchanges:　*1*　*Veg*

Cholesterol:　*0*　*Mg*
SF:　*<1*　*Gm*
Fat:　*<1*　*Gm*
Sodium:　*51*　*Mg*
Dietary Fiber:　*2*　*Gm*

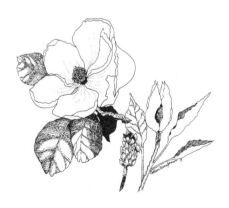

OLD FASHIONED BAKED BEANS

2 **cups dry navy beans**
2 **quarts water**
1 **cup chopped onion**
4 **ounces Healthy Choice smoked ham, cubed**
¾ **cup molasses**
1 **teaspoon salt**
1 **tablespoon yellow prepared mustard**

Rinse beans in cold water and drain. Place in large saucepan and add water. Bring to boil for 2 minutes. Remove from heat, cover and let stand for an hour. Return to heat and bring to a boil. Turn the burner to medium low and simmer for one hour. Drain beans and reserve liquid. Pour beans into a 2½ quart casserole. Add onion and ham. Mix lightly. Mix 2 cups of reserved bean liquid with molasses, salt and dry mustard. Pour over beans. Cover and bake in 300 degree F oven 5 - 6 hours. Check every hour after the second hour. The beans will start out covered with liquid and at the end, the beans should be very moist and coated with syrupy liquid.

Yield: 10 servings

Calories: 161
Exchanges: 1   Bread
*   ½   Veg*

Cholesterol: 6   Mg
SF: 0   Gm
Fat: <1   Gm
Sodium: 375 Mg
Dietary Fiber: 4   Gm

BROCCOLI CHEESE CASSEROLE

1¼ pounds frozen broccoli
1   can Healthy Request cream of mushroom soup
¼   teaspoon onion powder
¼   teaspoon salt
⅛   teaspoon garlic powder
⅛   teaspoon black pepper
1   4 ounce can sliced mushrooms drained
½   cup grated low-fat cheddar cheese

Thaw broccoli. Squeeze out excess moisture and set aside. In a large mixing bowl, combine soup, onion powder, garlic powder, pepper and mushrooms. Add broccoli spears. Place mixture in a 2 quart casserole that has been sprayed with cooking spray. Sprinkle cheese over the top. Bake at 350 degrees F for 30 - 35 minutes or until bubbly.

Yield: 8 servings

Calories: 73
Exchanges: *1   Meat*
          ½   Bread
          ½   Veg

Cholesterol: 11 Mg
SF: 2   Gm
Fat: 3   Gm
Sodium: 296 Mg
Dietary Fiber: <1 Gm

BROCCOLI CHEESE ROLL-UPS

2 **cups broccoli flowerettes, chopped**
2 **green chopped onions**
8 **lasagna noodles**
  vegetable cooking spray
1 **can Healthy Request cream of mushroom soup**
4 **ounces fat free Ricotta cheese**
½ **cup Parmesan cheese**

In a saucepan sauté onions in non-stick vegetable spray. Add 1 can of soup. Heat thoroughly and set aside. Combine cheeses in a small bowl. Set aside. Cook lasagna noodles until tender but firm. Drain well on a towel. Steam broccoli and squeeze out excess water. Mix broccoli and cheese in with half of the sauce mixture. Reserve half the sauce for later use. Spread 3 or 4 table-spoons of sauce mixture on each lasagna noodle. Roll each noodle up in jelly roll fashion. Place in a baking pan prepared with non-stick vegetable spray, seam side down. Pour remaining sauce over noodles. Bake covered for 15 minutes in a 325 degree F oven.

Yield: 8 servings

Calories: 127
Exchanges: *1* *Bread*
  ½ *Veg*

Cholesterol: *7* *Mg*
SF: *0* *Gm*
Fat: *<1* *Gm*
Sodium: *106 Mg*
Dietary Fiber: *1* *Gm*

BROCCOLI SOUFFLE

- **10** ounces frozen chopped broccoli
- **1** tablespoon dehydrated onion flakes
- **½** cup egg substitute
- **8** ounces fat free sour cream
- **1½** teaspoons cornstarch
- **1** tablespoon dry butter substitute granules
- **¼** teaspoon black pepper
- **2** ounces fat free cheddar cheese
- **¼** cups grated Parmesan cheese
  vegetable cooking spray

Thaw and drain chopped broccoli. Add egg beaters, onion and all other ingredients. Pour into 2 quart casserole that has been treated with cooking spray. Bake at 350 degrees F for 25 minutes or until center is set.

Yield: 4 servings

Calories: 118
Exchanges:	*2*	*Meat*
	1	*Veg*

Cholesterol:	*7*	*Mg*
SF:	*1*	*Gm*
Fat:	*2*	*Gm*
Sodium:	*347*	*Mg*
Dietary Fiber:	*2*	*Gm*

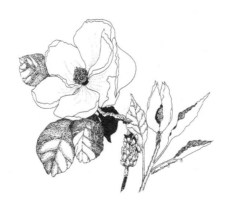

SUNSHINE CARROTS

4½ cups carrots
½ tablespoon fat free mayonnaise
2 tablespoons chopped onions
2 tablespoons prepared horseradish
¼ teaspoon salt
   dash of black pepper
1 serving Snackwell cheese crackers

Steam carrots about 10 minutes or until they are cooked to your preference. Drain. Combine mayonnaise, onion, horseradish, pepper. Toss with carrots. Place in a 1 quart casserole that has been sprayed with vegetable cooking spray. Crush crackers and spray crumbs with butter flavored cooking spray. Run under the broiler for about 1 - 2 minutes, only to ensure the crackers will remain crisp.

Yield: 6 servings

Calories: 79
Exchanges: *2   Veg*

Cholesterol: *0   Mg*
SF: *<1   Gm*
Fat: *1   Gm*
Sodium: *294 Mg*
Dietary Fiber: *5   Gm*

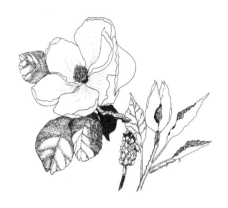

KAHLUA CARROTS

1 **pound carrots**
1 **tablespoon light margarine**
2 **tablespoons Kahlua**
1 **tablespoon brown sugar, packed**
   dash of salt

Scrape and slice carrots. Put into glass bowl. Add 2 tablespoons water. Cover and steam in microwave for 3 minutes on high. Set aside. Spray skillet with vegetable cooking spray. Melt 1 tablespoon light margarine. Add 1 tablespoon brown sugar and 2 tablespoons Kahlua. Cook until mixture boils. Add carrots. Toss and cook until just heated.

Yield: 6 servings

Calories: 63
Exchanges: *1 Veg*
          ½ Fruit

Cholesterol: *63 Mg*
SF: *<1 Gm*
Fat: *1 Gm*
Sodium: *110 Mg*
Dietary Fiber: *3 Gm*

CREAMY CAULIFLOWER

2 pounds raw cauliflower
2 slices white bread
2 cups nonfat skim milk
2 ounces liquid Butter Buds
8 ounces fat free American cheese
½ cup chopped onion
½ cup diced celery
dash of black pepper

Break slices of bread into pieces. Soak in milk for about 10 minutes. Add Butter Buds, onion and celery. Season to taste and cook over medium low heat until mixture thickens. In a separate uncovered saucepan, break cauliflower and cook 5 minutes in enough boiling water to cover it. Drain completely. Put cauliflower into 2 quart casserole. Add bread milk mixture. Cover with thin cheese slices and bake 350 degrees F until cheese melts, approximately 10 minutes.

Yield: 8 servings

Calories: 96
Exchanges: ½ *Meat*
1 *Veg*

Cholesterol: 1 *Mg*
SF: <1 *Gm*
Fat: <1 *Gm*
Sodium: 338 *Mg*
Dietary Fiber: 3 *Gm*

BRAISED CELERY IN CONSOMME

12	ribs of celery, cut in strips
½	cup chopped onion
4	cups sliced mushrooms
1	tablespoon dry butter substitute granules
10	ounces beef consomme
2	tablespoons grated Parmesan cheese

Scrub celery. Remove top leaves. Cut each rib lengthwise through the heart. Cut into desired lengths. Arrange celery on top of onions and mushrooms in a 2 quart casserole. Sprinkle with butter substitute and pepper. Add consomme and bake covered for 1 hour at 375 degrees F. Sprinkle with Parmesan cheese before serving.

Yield: 6 servings

Calories: 70
Exchanges: 2 *Veg*

Cholesterol: 2 *Mg*
SF: <1 *Gm*
Fat: <1 *Gm*
Sodium: 481 *Mg*
Dietary Fiber: 2 *Gm*

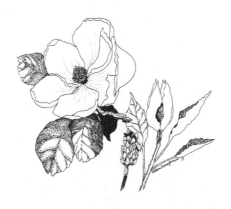

SCALLOPED CORN

1	can (17 ounces) cream corn
½	cup egg substitute
6	cups crushed saltines
¼	cup skim evaporated milk
4	teaspoons dry butter substitute
1	tablespoon minced celery
1	tablespoon minced onion
¼	cup shredded carrot
¼	cup minced bell pepper
⅛	teaspoon red pepper
½	cup shredded low fat cheddar cheese

Combine all ingredients except the cheese. Mix well. Pour into an 8" x 8" x 2" baking dish prepared with vegetable cooking spray. Top with cheese. Bake at 350 degrees F for 30 minutes.

Yield: 6 servings

Calories: 124
Exchanges: ½   Meat
*   1   Bread*

Cholesterol: 6   Mg
SF: 0   Gm
Fat: 2   Gm
Sodium: 114 Mg
Dietary Fiber: 1   Gm

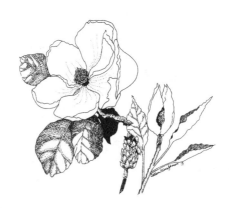

CORN CASSEROLE WITH TOMATOES

½ cup chopped bell pepper
½ cup chopped onion
¼ cup all purpose flour
1 16 ounce can of tomatoes, diced
3 16 ounce cans of corn, drained
2 egg whites, boiled
¼ teaspoon Tabasco sauce
¼ teaspoon black pepper
1 teaspoon Worcestershire sauce
4 ounces grated light Colby cheese
vegetable cooking spray

Sauté bell peppers and onions. Add flour and stir mix well. Set aside. Combine tomatoes and corn. Add to other vegetables. Stir in chopped egg whites and seasonings. Pour mixture into a casserole dish and bake 25 minutes at 350 degrees F. Sprinkle with cheese and bake another 3 to 5 minutes or until cheese melts.

Yield: 15 (¾ cup) servings

Calories: 86
Exchanges: *1*   *Bread*

Cholesterol: *5*   *Mg*
SF: *1*   *Gm*
Fat: *2*   *Gm*
Sodium: *308 Mg*
Dietary Fiber: *2*   *Gm*

CREOLE EGGPLANT

    4 cups eggplants, or 2 small eggplants
    1 cup fresh tomato, chopped
  1½ cups chopped onion
    4 ounces fat free cheddar cheese
    2 teaspoons baking powder
    ½ cup chopped bell pepper
    ¼ cup egg substitute
    2 ounces Canadian bacon, chopped
    ½ cup bread crumbs
    ¼ teaspoon black pepper

Peel and slice eggplants. Place in large pot and boil until tender. Drain and mash. Add egg, tomato, salt, cheese, onion and pepper to eggplant. Stir in baking powder and chopped Canadian bacon. Mix well and place in baking dish prepared with cooking spray. Sprinkle with bread crumbs and bake for 40 minutes at 350 degrees F.

Yield: 8 (½ cup) servings

Calories: 73
Exchanges: ½ *Meat*
                 1 *Veg*

Cholesterol: 5 *Mg*
SF: <1 *Gm*
Fat: 1 *Gm*
Sodium: 264 *Mg*
Dietary Fiber: 1 *Gm*

SOUTHERN GARDEN MEDLEY

2 **cups sliced raw summer squash**
2 **cups sliced zucchini squash**
1 **cup chopped onion**
1 **cup sliced tomato**
2 **tablespoons butter substitute granules**
2 **ounces light cheddar cheese**
1 **serving Snackwell cheese crackers**

In a 2 quart casserole, layer vegetables in the order they fall in the recipe. Sprinkle cheese and butter substitute throughout the layering. Crush cheese crackers and place on top of casserole. Bake at 350 degrees F for 30 minutes.

Yield: 6 servings

Calories: 84
Exchanges: 2 *Veg*

Cholesterol: 5 *Mg*
SF: <1 *Gm*
Fat: <1 *Gm*
Sodium: 251 *Mg*
Dietary Fiber: 2 *Gm*

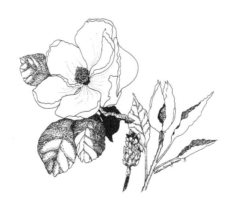

GARDEN PILAF

1   cup chopped onion
2   cloves of garlic
½   teaspoon red pepper
2   tablespoons balsamic vinegar
¼   teaspoon black pepper
2   cups broccoli flowerettes
1   cup sliced squash
½   cup diced carrots
4   cups long grain rice
2   tablespoons grated Parmesan cheese
1   can defatted chicken broth
    vegetable cooking spray

Cook rice in defatted chicken broth until "just" done. Do not overcook. Steam the broccoli, squash and carrots until "crunchy" done. Spray a large non-stick skillet with cooking spray. Over medium heat, cook onions, garlic and red pepper until onions are golden. Remove from heat. Stir in vinegar, black pepper, broccoli, squash, carrots and cooked rice. Toss to combine and sprinkle with Parmesan cheese.

Yield: 8 (1 cup) servings

Calories: 155
Exchanges: 1   *Bread*
                 1   *Veg*

Cholesterol: 3   *Mg*
SF: <1   *Gm*
Fat: 2   *Gm*
Sodium: 71   *Mg*
Dietary Fiber: 3   *Gm*

CHEESE GRITS

2 cups cooked grits
4 ounces skim evaporated milk
8 ounces fat free American cheese slices
½ cup egg substitute
2 tablespoons dry butter substitute
1 teaspoon garlic powder
   dash red pepper
2 tablespoons chopped chives
   vegetable cooking spray

In saucepan heat skim evaporated milk, butter substitute and cheese, stirring constantly until dissolved and mixed well. Pour cheese mixture into grits. Add egg substitute, garlic, red pepper and chives. Mix well and pour into a casserole dish prepared with non-stick vegetable spray. Bake at 350 degrees F for 30 to 40 minutes.

Yield: 8 servings

Calories: 87
Exchanges: ½ *Meat*
              1   *Bread*

Cholesterol: 5   *Mg*
SF: 0   *Gm*
Fat: 0   *Gm*
Sodium: 408 *Mg*
Dietary Fiber: 0   *Gm*

MUSHROOM RICE

1   cup long grain rice
2   cups chopped raw mushrooms
16   ounces fat free beef broth
1   ounce red wine
¼   teaspoon black pepper
1   tablespoon Molly McButter, sour cream flavor
2   tablespoons dehydrated onion flakes

Combine all ingredients. Bake in a 1½ quart casserole dish uncovered for 1 hour at 350 degrees F.

Yield: 8 servings

Calories: 103
Exchanges: *½ Bread*
               ½ Veg

Cholesterol: *0 Mg*
SF: *0 Gm*
Fat: *<1 Gm*
Sodium: *55 Mg*
Dietary Fiber: *<1 Gm*

CREAMY RICH NOODLES

8   ounces egg noodles
1   package dry Italian salad dressing
¼   cup evaporated skim milk
3   tablespoons dry butter substitute
2   tablespoons fresh grated Parmesan cheese

May use fat free Parmesan cheese.

Cook noodles as directed, omitting any oil. Drain well. Add remaining ingredients and lightly toss to blend thoroughly.

Yield: 8 (½ cup) servings

Calories: 135
Exchanges: *1 Bread*

Cholesterol: *29 Mg*
SF: *<1 Gm*
Fat: *2 Gm*
Sodium: *377 Mg*
Dietary Fiber: *0 Gm*

BAKED VIDALIA ONION

4   large Vidalia onions (any large sweet onion will do)
4   teaspoons dry butter substitute

Remove the outer skins and wash the onions. Wrap each onion in aluminum foil. Bake at 350 degrees F for 1 hour. Remove foil and sprinkle with the dry butter substitute.

Yield: 4 servings

Calories: 94
Exchanges: *2   Veg*

Cholesterol: *0   Mg*
SF: *0   Gm*
Fat: *<1 Gm*
Sodium: *65 Mg*
Dietary Fiber: *2   Gm*

CHEESY SWEET ONIONS

2   pounds onions, sliced
½   cup water
2   tablespoons dry butter substitute
1   cup skim evaporated milk
½   cup light cheddar cheese
2   tablespoons vermouth
¼   teaspoon paprika
3   tablespoons cornstarch

Slice 2 very large sweet onions (Texas sweet or Vidalia). About 2 pounds. Combine onions and water into a 2 quart covered casserole. Cover and microwave about 4 minutes on high. Drain onions, and place in a baking pan. Reserve liquid. Mix cornstarch, milk, vermouth and ½ cup onion stock. Pour over onions. Sprinkle with cheese and paprika. Place uncovered in a 350 degree F oven for 25 - 30 minutes or until mixture is bubbling and sauce has thickened.

Yield: 6 servings

Calories: 140
Exchanges: *2   Veg*
                 ½   Milk

Cholesterol: *7   Mg*
SF: *1   Gm*
Fat: *2   Gm*
Sodium: *242 Mg*
Dietary Fiber: *3   Gm*

SPICY FIELD PEAS

1	pound field peas
1	cup water
2	ounces Healthy Choice ham
1	cup onion, chopped
1	clove garlic
½	teaspoon salt
1	teaspoon cumin
⅛	teaspoon dry mustard
1	teaspoon chili powder
1	teaspoon black pepper
1	ounce fresh parsley
1	teaspoon liquid smoke
1	can (16 ounces) stewed tomatoes

Shell peas. Wash and pick. Drain. Put all ingredients into a large saucepan and bring to a boil. Reduce heat to a simmer. Cook about 1 hour.

Peas and rice or peas and cornbread will give a complete protein when eaten at the same meal.

Yield: 6 (¾ cup) servings

Calories: 128
Exchanges: *1*   *Bread*
                 1   *Veg*

Cholesterol: *4*   *Mg*
SF: *<1* *Gm*
Fat: *1*   *Gm*
Sodium: *468 Mg*
Dietary Fiber: *7*   *Gm*

OVEN FRIES

1 **large sliced raw potato**
1 **egg white**
2 **tablespoons fat free Parmesan cheese**
2 **tablespoons all purpose flour**
  vegetable cooking spray

Cut a potato lengthwise into wedges. Toss with beaten egg white. Sprinkle with Parmesan cheese and flour. Place on baking pan prepared with non-stick vegetable spray. Spray potatoes with non-stick vegetable spray. Bake at 425 degrees F for 25 minutes.

Yield: 2 servings

Calories: 194
Exchanges: 2   *Bread*

Cholesterol: 41 *Mg*
SF: 0 *Gm*
Fat: <1 *Gm*
Sodium: 80 *Mg*
Dietary Fiber: 3 *Gm*

PLEATED BAKED POTATOES

6 **baking potatoes**
½ **cup liquid Butter Buds**
1 **tablespoon chopped fresh chives**
½ **teaspoon black pepper**

Wash potatoes and dry. Cut each potato crosswise into ⅛" slices, into, but not through to the bottom of each potato. Place on baking sheet prepared with vegetable cooking spray. Combine liquid butter substitute and seasonings. Brush over potatoes. Bake for 1 hour or until done at 400 degrees F.

Yield: 6 servings

Calories: 154
Exchanges: 2   *Bread*

Cholesterol: 0 *Mg*
SF: 0 *Gm*
Fat: <1 *Gm*
Sodium: 245 *Mg*
Dietary Fiber: 4 *Gm*

TWICE BAKED POTATOES

6 baking potatoes
2 ounces liquid Butter Buds
8 ounces light cheddar cheese
8 ounces fat free sour cream
4 chopped green onions
¼ teaspoon black pepper
¼ cup evaporated skim milk
   butter flavored cooking spray

Bake potatoes at 400 degrees F for 1 hour or until done. In a microwave safe saucepan, combine liquid Butter Buds and cheese. Heat until almost melted, about 1 minute. Remove from microwave. Blend in sour cream, onions and pepper. Cut baked potatoes in half lengthwise and scoop out the pulp. Place in a large bowl and mash. Fold cheese mixture into the mashed potatoes. Stuff potato skins. Spray with butter flavored cooking spray. Bake in a 350 degree F oven for 10 minutes. Great to serve with grilled chicken, steamed vegetable and a green salad.

Yield: 12 servings

Calories: 164
Exchanges: ½ *Meat*
          1½ *Bread*

Cholesterol: 10 *Mg*
SF: 1   *Gm*
Fat: 3   *Gm*
Sodium: 340 *Mg*
Dietary Fiber: 3   *Gm*

BROCCOLI-CHEESE POTATOES

4   baked potatoes
½   cup skimmed milk
¼   teaspoon onion powder
¼   teaspoon garlic powder
    dash of black pepper
1   package frozen chopped broccoli, boiled
½   cup grated fat free cheese
    dash of paprika
1   tablespoon Parmesan cheese

Cut potatoes in half lengthwise and scoop out the insides. Place the potato pulp, milk, onion powder, garlic powder and pepper in a large bowl. Mix potatoes with a hand mixer until smooth and creamy. Stir in broccoli and cheese. Divide this mixture and place back into the potato skins. Sprinkle with paprika and Parmesan cheese. Put potatoes on baking sheet. Bake at 400 degrees F until lightly brown.

Yield: 8 servings

Calories: 153
Exchanges: ½ *Meat*
                1 *Bread*

Cholesterol: 4 *Mg*
SF: 0 *Gm*
Fat: 1 *Gm*
Sodium: 151 *Mg*
Dietary Fiber: 4 *Gm*

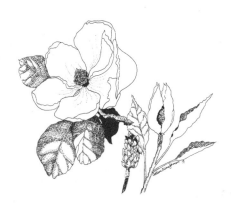

CREAMED NEW POTATOES

3 pounds new potatoes
1½ cups skim milk
3 tablespoons cornstarch
2 teaspoons onion flakes
⅓ teaspoon black pepper
2 tablespoons dry butter substitute

Wash and peel about 3 pounds of new potatoes. Put into saucepan and cover with water. Boil about 15 minutes or until potatoes are tender. Drain and set aside. In saucepan mix milk, onion flakes, cornstarch and black pepper. Bring to a boil. Allow to boil about 3 minutes over medium heat, stirring constantly. Add potatoes. Sprinkle with butter substitute and coat with sauce.

Yield: 8 servings

Calories: 165
Exchanges: *2*   *Bread*

Cholesterol: *1*   *Mg*
SF: *0*   *Gm*
Fat: *0*   *Gm*
Sodium: *79*   *Mg*
Dietary Fiber: *3*   *Gm*

OLD FASHIONED WHIPPED POTATOES

2 pounds potatoes
¼ cup non fat dried milk
3 tablespoons dry butter substitute granules
¼ teaspoon salt

Peel and quarter potatoes. Put into saucepan and cover with water. Add salt. Bring to a boil. Cook about 20 minutes. Drain. Reserve about 2 cups of potato stock. Beat potatoes with an electric mixer. Add non fat powdered milk, butter substitute and enough potato stock to get the desired consistency.

Yield: 6 (½ cup) servings

Calories: 144
Exchanges: *2*   *Bread*

Cholesterol: *1*   *Mg*
SF: *0*   *Gm*
Fat: *0*   *Gm*
Sodium: *250*   *Mg*
Dietary Fiber: *1*   *Gm*

SWEET POTATO SURPRISE

2 **large sweet potatoes**
⅔ **cup sugar**
2 **tablespoons light margarine**
2 **tablespoons dry butter substitute**
1 **cup egg substitute**
1 **teaspoon vanilla**
1 **cup marshmallows**
   vegetable cooking spray

Peel and boil potatoes. Drain and mash. Mix potatoes, sugar, margarine, butter substitute, egg substitute, vanilla and salt. Place in casserole that has been sprayed with cooking spray. Place marshmallows on top of potato mixture. Bake at 350 degrees F until casserole is set and marshmallows are browned (about 30 minutes).

Yield: 9 servings

Calories: 178
Exchanges: Not acceptable for diabetics.

Cholesterol: *0   Mg*
SF: *<1 Gm*
Fat: *2   Gm*
Sodium: *99 Mg*
Dietary Fiber: *2   Gm*

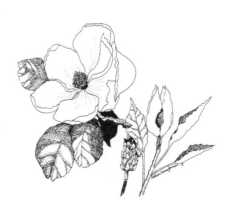

SPINACH CASSEROLE

30 ounces frozen spinach, chopped
 8 ounces Healthy Choice fat free cream cheese
    (herb/garlic)
 2 egg whites
10 ounces Campbell's Healthy Request cream of
    mushroom soup
 2 ounces Parmesan cheese, grated
 3 ounces canned fried onion rings

Separate eggs and throw away egg yolks. Beat egg whites until they hold a peak, set aside. Heat soup, stir in cream cheese until it becomes creamy. Add thawed, drained spinach (squeeze between paper towels to remove all moisture). Fold in beaten egg whites and Parmesan cheese. Pour into casserole. Top with onion rings and bake at 350 degrees F for 35 minutes.

Yield: 12 servings

Calories: 86
Exchanges: *1*   *Meat*
                 ½ *Veg*

Cholesterol: *8*   *Mg*
SF: *<1* *Gm*
Fat: *3*   *Gm*
Sodium: *349* *Mg*
Dietary Fiber: *2*   *Gm*

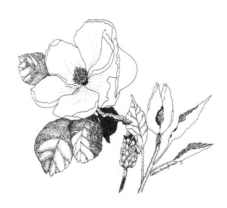

SQUASH CASSEROLE

CORNBREAD:

¼ cup egg substitute
½ cup cornmeal
½ cup all purpose flour
2 teaspoons baking powder
½ cup skim milk
   vegetable cooking spray

CASSEROLE:

½ cup egg substitute
2 cups sliced squash, boiled and drained
½ cup butter substitute granules
1 cup chopped onions
1 10 ounce can Campbell's Healthy Request cream of chicken soup
1 cup grated light cheddar cheese
   dash of pepper

Make cornbread by mixing the cornmeal, flour and baking powder. Add milk and egg substitute. Beat until smooth. Bake in small skillet prepared with non-stick vegetable spray at 425 degrees F for 20 minutes or until done. Next, cook onion in non-stick spray until clear. Crumble cornbread into drained cooked squash, adding soup and slightly beaten egg substitute. Season with pepper. Top with cheese. Bake at 350 degrees F for 30 minutes or until bubbles well.

Yield: 8 servings

Calories: 175
Exchanges: 1½ *Meat*
        1 *Bread*

Cholesterol: 16 *Mg*
SF: 2 *Gm*
Fat: 5 *Gm*
Sodium: 680 *Mg*
Dietary Fiber: 2 *Gm*

DILLED YELLOW SQUASH

3   pounds sliced summer squash
1   cup chopped onions
2   tablespoon butter substitute granules
8   ounces fat free sour cream
1½ tablespoons dried dill weed
⅛   teaspoon salt
¼   teaspoon black pepper
1   serving Snackwell cheese crackers
    butter flavored cooking spray

Place slice squash in a small amount of water with onion. Cook until tender. Drain well. Mash squash and onion. Add butter substitute, sour cream, dill weed, salt and pepper. Pour into a 3 quart casserole. Top with crushed cheese crackers and spray with butter flavored cooking spray. Bake at 325 degrees F for 20 to 30 minutes.

Yield: 8 servings

Calories: 70
Exchanges: *2   Veg*

Cholesterol: *0   Mg*
SF: *<1   Gm*
Fat: *1   Gm*
Sodium: *140 Mg*
Dietary Fiber: *3   Gm*

TURNIP GREENS WITH TURNIPS

1 **pound turnip greens, fresh or frozen**
4 **ounces Healthy Choice ham**
2 **cups diced turnips**
1 **teaspoon sugar**
½ **teaspoon salt**
1 **teaspoon liquid smoke**
4 **cups water**

Put all ingredients into large saucepan. Bring to a boil. Reduce heat and simmer 45 minutes to an hour.

Yield: 6 servings

Calories: 57
Exchanges: *½   Meat*
                      1   Veg

Cholesterol: 10 Mg
SF: <1 Gm
Fat: 1   Gm
Sodium: 387 Mg
Dietary Fiber: 3   Gm

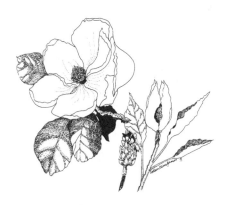

VEGETABLE BUNDLES

olive oil flavored cooking spray
2 cups raw chopped broccoli
½ cup chopped red bell peppers
1 cup chopped green onions
1 cup canned white beans, drained and washed
2 tablespoons low salt soy sauce
12 sheets phyllo dough (9" x 13")
2 tablespoons extra light margarine

Spray skillet with non-stick vegetable spray. Add broccoli, peppers and onions. Cook until vegetables are tender but crisp. Remove skillet from heat. Stir in the beans, seasonings and soy sauce. Set aside. Place the sheets of phyllo in a stack on a piece of waxed paper. Cover with plastic wrap, then a damp kitchen towel to prevent drying. Take 2 sheets of the phyllo and place on another piece of waxed paper. Brush with light margarine. Then, top with 2 more sheets of phyllo and brush with margarine. Using a sharp knife, cut the buttered stack into 4 squares. Place ¼ cup vegetable filling in the center of each square. Bring the 4 corners up together, pinch and twist slightly. Place each bundle as assembled in a non-stick muffin tin. Repeat assembling bundles until balance of ingredients have been used. Bake at 375 degrees F until brown.

Yield: 12 servings

Calories: 125
Exchanges: *1½ Bread*
                       ½ Fat

Cholesterol: *0   Mg*
SF: *0   Gm*
Fat: *3   Gm*
Sodium: *207 Mg*
Dietary Fiber: *3   Gm*

VEGETABLES FOR A CROWD

2 10 ounce packages chopped broccoli
1 10 ounce package chopped spinach
10 ounces frozen artichoke hearts
2 cups sliced zucchini squash
1 cup grated Parmesan cheese
8 ounces sliced raw mushrooms
1 tablespoon dry butter substitute granules
¼ teaspoon black pepper
½ teaspoon ground oregano
¼ teaspoon garlic powder
4 cups egg substitute
2 tablespoons dehydrated onion flakes
   vegetable cooking spray

Thaw and drain all frozen vegetables. Add remaining ingredients except egg substitute. Just before baking, mix egg substitute with vegetables. Pour into a 13" x 9" pan that has been sprayed with cooking spray. Bake uncovered at 350 degrees F for 35 - 40 minutes.

Yield: 16 servings

Calories: 72
Exchanges: *½ Meat*
                  1 Veg

Cholesterol: *5 Mg*
SF: *1 Gm*
Fat: *2 Gm*
Sodium: *209 Mg*
Dietary Fiber: *3 Gm*

VEGETABLE VERMICELLI

vegetable cooking spray
2 cups raw chopped broccoli
1 cup chopped green peppers
2 cloves of garlic
16 ounces canned stewed tomatoes
10 ounces frozen artichoke hearts, thawed
½ cup pimiento
6 slices sun dried tomato slices
1 teaspoon ground basil
1 teaspoon ground oregano
⅛ teaspoon crush red pepper
12 ounces vermicelli

Cook vermicelli according to package directions, excluding any oil. In a large skillet coated with non-stick vegetable cooking spray, add broccoli, green peppers and garlic. Cook, stirring frequently until they are crisp but tender (2 - 3 minutes). Stir in stewed tomatoes, artichokes, sun dried tomatoes, pimientos, basil, oregano and red pepper. Bring to a boil over high heat. Reduce heat to low. Partially cover and simmer until sauce thickens (20 - 25 minutes). Toss vegetables with hot vermicelli and serve.

Yield: 6 servings (1 cup vermicelli plus ¾ cup sauce)

Calories: 321
Exchanges: *2½ Bread*
                 4 Veg

Cholesterol: *0 Mg*
SF: *<1 Gm*
Fat: *2 Gm*
Sodium: *335 Mg*
Dietary Fiber: *7 Gm*

VEGETABLE PICANTE

1   pound sliced zucchini squash
2   cups raw chopped eggplant
1   cup chopped onion
½   cup chopped bell peppers
1   can (8 ounces) picante sauce
1   small can (6 ounces) tomato paste
¼   teaspoon black pepper

Combine first 5 ingredients. Bring to a boil, simmer covered for 30 minutes or until tender. Stir in tomato paste and seasonings. Reheat slowly to blend flavors. Serve hot as a side dish or chill and serve cold with baked tortilla chip or pita chips as an appetizer.

Yield: 38 servings

Calories: 8
Exchanges: *2   Veg*

Cholesterol: *0   Mg*
SF: *<1   Gm*
Fat: *1   Gm*
Sodium: *448   Mg*
Dietary Fiber: *2   Gm*

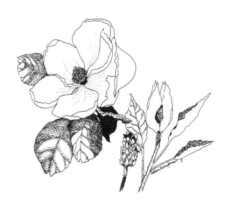

SUMMER'S DELIGHT

1   chopped bell pepper
6   sliced tomatoes
2   teaspoons dry garlic and herbs salad dressing
¼   teaspoon black pepper
¼   teaspoon red pepper
1   tablespoon brown sugar
3   green onions, chopped
1   cup dry bread crumbs
4   ounces liquid Butter Buds
2   ounces light cheddar cheese, shredded
     vegetable cooking spray

Spray a 2 quart casserole with cooking spray. Begin by peeling and slicing tomatoes into ½" slices. (An easy way to peel tomatoes is to dip tomatoes into boiling water for 15 seconds). After dipping, the skin will easily slip off. Mix all seasonings. Season while stacking tomatoes, add bell peppers. Pour Butter Buds over entire mixture. Top with onions, bread crumbs and cheese. Bake at 375 degrees F for 25 minutes.

Yield: 8 servings

Calories: 123
Exchanges: *1   Bread*
              2   Veg

Cholesterol: *4   Mg*
SF: *<1 Gm*
Fat: *2   Gm*
Sodium: *710 Mg*
Dietary Fiber: *2   Gm*

SWEET AND SOUR VEGETABLES

2 tablespoons sweet and sour marinade
2 tablespoons water
½ ounce vermouth
  vegetable cooking spray
2 green chopped onions
1 cup chopped broccoli
2 mushrooms, sliced
1 cup cauliflower, chopped

Refer to index for Sweet and Sour Marinade. Blend all liquids. Spray skillet with cooking spray. Heat and add vegetables. Stir fry, stirring constantly, until green onions begin to wilt. This will take about 2 - 3 minutes. Quickly add liquid mixture. It will bubble. Serve hot. An excellent choice as side dish to any meat.

Yield: 4 servings

Calories: 27
Exchanges: *1*   *Veg*

Cholesterol: *0*   *Mg*
SF: *0*   *Gm*
Fat: *<1*   *Gm*
Sodium: *146* *Mg*
Dietary Fiber: *1*   *Gm*

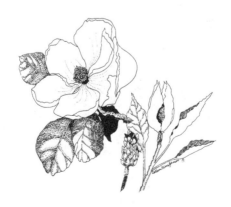

QUICK ZUCCHINI AND RED SAUCE

1 cup chopped onion
3 cups raw zucchini, sliced
1 cup raw yellow squash, sliced
2 cloves garlic
½ teaspoon oregano
1 cup fat free spaghetti sauce

Spray a large skillet with non-stick vegetable spray. Sauté onion, zucchini, yellow squash and garlic until vegetables are tender. Add oregano and nonfat spaghetti sauce. Cover and cook on low heat until heated thoroughly.

Yield: 8 servings

Calories: 33
Exchanges: 1   Veg

Cholesterol: 0   Mg
SF: 0   Gm
Fat: <1   Gm
Sodium: 212   Mg
Dietary Fiber: 2   Gm

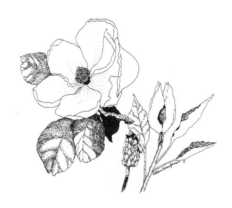

BREADS

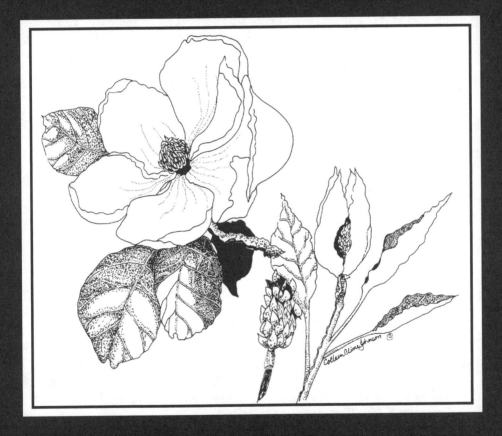

BREAKFAST BISCUITS

　　　vegetable cooking spray
½　pound Canadian bacon
1　cup all purpose flour
4　ounces fat free cheddar cheese
2　teaspoons baking powder
⅛　teaspoon red or cayenne pepper
1　cup evaporated skim canned milk

Sauté chopped Canadian bacon in cooking spray for 2 or 3 minutes. Combine bacon, flour and next 3 ingredients in a bowl. Add milk, stirring until dry ingredients are moistened. Drop by heaping tablespoons onto a baking sheet prepared with cooking spray. Bake at 400 degrees F for 22 minutes.

Yield: 12 servings

Calories 115
Exchanges:　　*1　Meat*
　　　　　　　1　Bread

Cholesterol:　　*2　Mg*
SF:　　　　　*0　Gm*
Fat:　　　　　*3　Gm*
Sodium　　　*248 Mg*
Dietary Fiber:　*<1　Gm*

SOUR CREAM BISCUITS

2　cups self rising flour
1　cup fat free sour cream
½　cup club soda

Combine ingredients. Stir with a fork until blended. Turn dough out onto a lightly floured surface and knead 10 - 12 times. Roll dough to ½" thickness. Cut with a 1" biscuit cutter. Place on a lightly greased baking sheet. Bake at 450 degrees F 10 - 12 minutes.

Yield: 1 dozen biscuits

Calories: 84
Exchanges:　　*1　Bread*

Cholesterol:　　*0　Mg*
SF:　　　　　*20　Gm*
Fat:　　　　　*<1　Gm*
Sodium:　　　*274 Mg*
Dietary Fiber:　*1　Gm*

BEER BREAD

2 cups all purpose flour
1½ cups whole wheat flour
1 teaspoon baking powder
3 tablespoons sugar
½ teaspoon salt
1 can light beer
¼ cup egg substitute
butter flavored spray

In a mixing bowl, combine dry ingredients. Make a well in the center of mixture. Add beer and egg substitute. Stir until ingredients are moistened. Spoon batter into a loaf pan that has been coated with cooking spray. Bake at 375 degrees F for 45 - 50 minutes or until a toothpick comes out clean. Let cool in pan for 10 minutes. Remove from pan. Cool on a wire rack.

Yield: 16 servings

Calories: 110
Exchanges: *1½ Bread*

Cholesterol: *0* *Mg*
SF: *0* *Gm*
Fat: *<1* *Gm*
Sodium: *128 Mg*
Dietary Fiber: *2* *Gm*

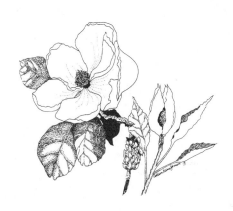

BREAKFAST BREAD

2½ cups 40% bran flakes
½ cup hot water
3 tablespoons stick margarine
1½ cups all purpose flour
1 teaspoon baking powder
1 teaspoon baking soda
⅓ cup brown sugar, packed
½ teaspoon cinnamon
1 cup non fat buttermilk
¼ cup egg substitute
½ cup seedless raisins
  vegetable cooking spray

Combine 1½ cups bran flakes, hot water and margarine in small bowl. Set aside. Combine remaining dry ingredients in large bowl. Make a well in the center of mixture and pour in buttermilk and egg substitute. Stir until moistened. Stir in cereal mixture and remaining bran flakes and raisins. Spoon into loaf pan coated with vegetable cooking spray. Bake at 350 degrees F for 55 minutes or until toothpick inserted comes out clean. Cool on a wire rack.

Yield: 16 servings

Calories: 111
Exchanges: Not acceptable for diabetics.

Cholesterol: *<1 Gm*
Fat: *1 Gm*
Sodium: *186 Mg*
Dietary Fiber: *2 Gm*

CRANBERRY CHRISTMAS BREAD

1½   cups cranberries, raw
  2   cups all purpose flour
  1   cup sugar
1½   teaspoons baking powder
  ½   teaspoon baking soda
  1   teaspoon salt
  ¼   cup lite stick margarine
  ¼   cup egg substitute
  ¾   cup orange juice
1½   cups golden seedless raisins

Wash cranberries, drain and grind in food processor until coarsely chopped. Set aside. Combine flour, sugar, baking powder, soda and salt in large mixing bowl. Cut in margarine with a pastry blender until margarine resembles coarse meal. Add egg substitute and orange juice. Stir in raisins and cranberries. Pour into pan prepared with cooking spray. Bake at 350 degrees F for 1 hour. Cool on wire rack.

Yield: 16 servings

Calories: 177
Exchanges: 2   *Bread*
              1   *Fruit*

Cholesterol: 0   *Mg*
SF: <1 *Gm*
Fat: 2   *Gm*
Sodium: 228 *Mg*
Dietary Fiber: 1   *Gm*

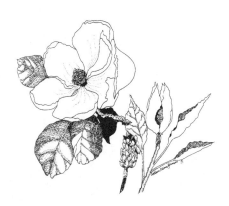

BRAIDED FRENCH BREAD

3 cups white bread flour
1 cup warm water
1 package dry yeast
1½ teaspoons salt
1 tablespoon cornmeal
   butter flavored cooking spray

Combine yeast with warm water. Let stand for 5 minutes. Blend flour and salt. Mix with liquid and knead 10 minutes. Place dough in bowl prepared with vegetable cooking spray. Cover and allow to rise free from drafts about 45 minutes. Spray baking pan with vegetable cooking spray. Sprinkle with cornmeal. Set aside. Punch down. Divide dough into 3 equal portions. Roll out into rectangles and roll up and seal. Pinch the 3 rolls together at one end and braid. Seal the end of the braid by pinching again. Place braid on baking pan. Spray with butter flavored cooking spray. Bake at 375 degrees F for 25 - 30 minutes.

Yield: 12 slices

Calories: 128
Exchanges: *1½ Bread*

Cholesterol: *0*   *Mg*
SF: *0*   *Gm*
Fat: *0*   *Gm*
Sodium: *268 Mg*
Dietary Fiber: *1*   *Gm*

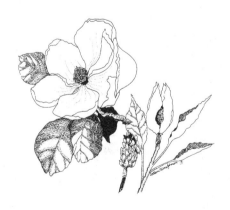

GARLIC BREAD STICKS

10 ounces refrigerated pizza dough
 1 egg white
 1 tablespoon water
 ¼ cup fat free Parmesan cheese
 ¼ teaspoon garlic powder
 1 ounce sesame seeds
 1 teaspoon dry butter substitute
   butter flavored cooking spray

Prepare sheet with cooking spray. Remove dough from package, but do not unroll. Cut dough into 12 slices. Unroll each slice. Cut in half and twist. Place on baking sheet. Mix egg white, water, dry butter substitute and garlic in small bowl. Baste each bread stick with egg white/liquid mixture. Sprinkle with fat free Parmesan and sesame seeds. Spray with cooking spray. Bake at 375 degrees F for 15 minutes or until brown.

Yield: 24 bread sticks

Calories: 41
Exchanges: *½* *Bread*
        ½ *Fat*

Cholesterol: *1*   *Mg*
SF: *<1* *Gm*
Fat: *1*   *Gm*
Sodium: *67* *Mg*
Dietary Fiber: *<1* *Gm*

SOFT PRETZELS

	vegetable cooking spray
1	package yeast
1½	cups water
½	teaspoon salt
1	tablespoon sugar
4	cups bread flour
¼	cup egg substitute
1	tablespoon coarse salt

Dissolve yeast in water with sugar. Add table salt and flour to yeast mixture. Mix to form a ball. Tear off pieces of dough and knead on floured board so they are not sticky. Form into desired shapes. Place on baking pan prepared with cooking spray. Brush with egg substitute. Sprinkle with coarse salt. Bake in 375 degree F oven for 10 - 15 minutes or until golden brown. Fun for kids to make.

Yield: 14

Calories: 148
Exchanges: *2   Bread*

Cholesterol: *0   Mg*
SF: *0   Gm*
Fat: *0   Gm*
Sodium: *236 Mg*
Dietary Fiber: *0   Gm*

AUNT ERA'S DUMPLINGS

1½ cups all purpose flour
½ teaspoon salt
   dash of pepper
1¾ cups water
2 cans (32 ounces) fat free chicken broth

Mix all ingredients except chicken broth in a bowl. Use hands. Knead dough. Make sure the flour is well mixed. Take half of mixture and put on floured waxed paper. Flatten with hands and sprinkle about 1 teaspoon over the flour mixture. Roll out thin. Cut into 1" squares.

Use more flour if squares seem to stick to the waxed paper. Set aside and repeat the same procedure with remaining dough. Let squares cool to room temperature. Drop squares into boiling chicken broth seasoned with salt and pepper. Use a spoon to move dumplings around so they won't stick to the bottom of the boiler. Let dumplings boil until they rise to the top. Turn off heat and cover. Allow to sit for 15 minutes.

Yield: 8 servings

Calories: 97
Exchanges: 1   Bread

Cholesterol: 0   Mg
SF: <1 Gm
Fat: 1   Gm
Sodium: 313 Mg

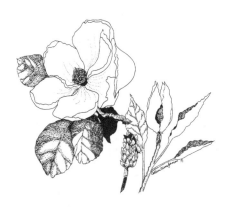

SOURDOUGH STARTER

1   package yeast
1   cup water
2   cups all purpose flour
3   tablespoons sugar
¾   teaspoon salt
2   cups water

STARTER:

Dissolve yeast in 1 cup warm water. Let stand 5 minutes. Combine flour, sugar and salt in a medium sized non-metal bowl. Stir well. Gradually stir in 2 cups warm water. Cover starter with cheese cloth. Let stand in a warm place for 72 hours. Stir 2 times a day. Place starter in refrigerator and stir once a day. Use within 11 days. When ready to use starter, take from refrigerator. Let stand at room temperature at least 1 hour. Stir and measure amount of starter needed for recipe. Replenish remainder starter with starter food (see below) and return to refrigerator.

STARTER FOOD:

½   cup sugar
1   cup all purpose flour
1   cup milk

Mix ingredients well. Stir into remaining sourdough starter.

Yield: 3 cups

SOURDOUGH BISCUITS

2 **cups self rising flour**
1 **teaspoon soda**
2 **tablespoons light margarine**
¼ **cup dry butter substitute granules**
¾ **cup sour dough starter**
½ **cup plus 1 tablespoon buttermilk made with skim milk**
  vegetable cooking spray

You may make buttermilk by combining ½ cup of skim milk and 1 table-spoon of vinegar and let sit for 2 minutes.

Combine flour and baking soda in a non-metal bowl. Stir Well. Cut in marga-rine with a fork or a pastry blender until mixture resembles coarse meal. Add sourdough starter and buttermilk. Stir until dry ingredients are moistened. Turn dough out onto a floured surface. Knead lightly 10 - 12 times. Roll dough to ½" thickness. Cut with a 2¾" biscuit cutter. Place on baking sheet that has been lightly sprayed with cooking spray.

Yield: 10 biscuits

Calories: 133
Exchanges: 1½ Bread

Cholesterol: <1 Mg
SF: <1 Gm
Fat: 2 Gm
Sodium: 228 Mg
Dietary Fiber: 1 Gm

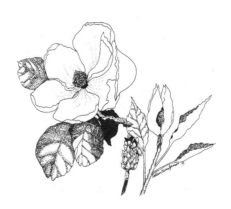

SOURDOUGH BUTTERMILK PANCAKES

2	cups all purpose flour
1½	teaspoons baking powder
½	teaspoon baking soda
½	teaspoon salt
2	tablespoons sugar
1½	cups buttermilk made with skim milk
1	cup sourdough starter
¼	cup egg substitute
2	tablespoons applesauce

You may make buttermilk by combining 1⅓ cups of skim milk and 2⅓ tablespoons of vinegar and let sit for 2 minutes.

Combine first 5 ingredients in a non-metal bowl. Stir well. Add buttermilk, sourdough starter and egg substitute. Beat only until large lumps disappear. Stir in applesauce. For each pancake pour about ¼ cup of batter on to a hot griddle sprayed with cooking spray. It may be necessary to spray griddle after each pancake.

Yield: 12 (4" pancakes)

Calories: 180
Exchanges: *1 Bread*

Cholesterol: *<1 Mg*
SF: *<1 Gm*
Fat: *<1 Gm*
Sodium: *180 Mg*
Dietary Fiber: *1 Gm*

CORNBREAD

vegetable cooking spray
1 cup all purpose flour
1 cup frozen whole kernel corn
1 cup cornmeal
2 tablespoons sugar
2 teaspoons baking powder
½ teaspoon salt
¼ teaspoon red pepper
1 cup skim milk
1 egg

Coat a 9" cast iron skillet with non-stick vegetable spray. Combine all ingredients, mixing well. Bake at 425 degrees F for 25 minutes or until wooden pick inserted in center comes out clean. Cut into wedges.

Yield: 12 servings

Calories: 129
Exchanges: *1½ Bread*

Cholesterol: *22 Mg*
SF: *<1 Gm*
Fat: *2 Gm*
Sodium: *157 Mg*
Dietary Fiber: *1 Gm*

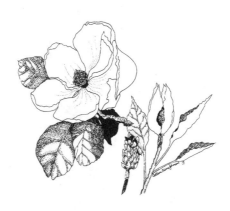

SPINACH CORNBREAD

1 box Jiffy cornbread mix
1 cup chopped onions
6 ounces fat free cottage cheese
4 ounces liquid Butter Buds
½ cup egg substitute
1 cup frozen spinach, chopped
vegetable cooking spray

Drain and press water from frozen chopped spinach. Combine spinach, onion, cottage cheese, butter substitute and egg substitute. Mix well. Add cornbread mix. Stir until all ingredients are thoroughly mixed. Pour into a skillet prepared with cooking spray. Spray top of raw cornbread with cooking spray. Bake at 400 degrees F for 25 minutes.

Yield: 12 servings

Calories: 173
Exchanges: ½ *Meat*
1½ *Bread*

Cholesterol: 1 *Mg*
SF: <1 *Gm*
Fat: 4 *Gm*
Sodium: 652 *Mg*
Dietary Fiber: 1 *Gm*

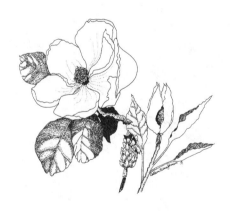

BASIC MUFFIN MIX

ONE RECIPE AMOUNT:

1½ cups white bread flour
½ cup sugar
2 teaspoons baking powder
½ teaspoon salt

BATCH RECIPE FOR MUFFIN MIX:

5 pounds white bread flour
6 cups sugar
3 tablespoons baking powder
2 tablespoons salt

You may store large amounts of the dry ingredients in an airtight container. This will keep several months in a cabinet and longer if kept in the refrigerator. See the following pages for various recipes with this mix.

APPLE MUFFINS

2 cups basic muffin mix
¼ cup egg substitute
½ cup skim milk
⅓ cup applesauce, unsweetened
3 cups chopped apples with skin
1 teaspoon cinnamon

Mix all ingredients, except apples Do not overbeat. Fold in apples. Fill muffin tins prepared with vegetable cooking spray or paper liners ⅔ full. Bake at 400 degrees F for 20 - 25 minutes.

Yield: 12 servings

Calories: 120
Exchanges: *1   Bread*
                 ½   Fruit

Cholesterol: *<1 Mg*
SF: *0   Gm*
Fat: *<1 Gm*
Sodium: *181 Mg*
Dietary Fiber: *1   Gm*

BLUEBERRY MUFFINS

> 2 cups basic muffin mix
> ¼ cup egg substitute
> ½ cup skim milk
> ⅓ cup applesauce, unsweetened
> ¾ cup blueberries, fresh or frozen, well drained

Mix all ingredients, except blueberries Do not overbeat. Fold in blueberries Fill muffin tins prepared with vegetable cooking spray or paper liners ⅔ full. Bake at 400 degrees F for 20 - 25 minutes

Yield: 12 servings

Calories: 108
Exchanges: *1*   *Bread*

Cholesterol: *24 Mg*
SF: *0   Gm*
Fat: *<1 Gm*
Sodium: *152 Mg*
Dietary Fiber: *1   Gm*

EASY MUFFINS

> 2 cups basic muffin mix
> ¼ cup egg substitute
> ½ cup skim milk
> ⅓ cup applesauce, unsweetened

Mix all ingredients. Do not overbeat. Fill muffin tins prepared with vegetable cooking spray or paper liners ⅔ full. Bake at 400 degrees F for 20 - 25 minutes.

Yield: 12 servings

Calories: 124
Exchanges: *1*   *Bread*

Cholesterol: *0   Mg*
SF: *0   Gm*
Fat: *<1 Gm*
Sodium: *181 Mg*
Dietary Fiber: *1   Gm*

JAM MUFFINS

2 cups basic muffin mix
¼ cup egg substitute
½ cup skim milk
⅓ cup applesauce, unsweetened
2 tablespoons jam or preserves

Mix all ingredients, except jam. Do not overbeat. Fill muffin tins prepared with vegetable cooking spray or paper liners ⅓ full. Top with ½ teaspoon jam or preserves. Spoon enough batter over top of preserves to leave each ⅔ full. Bake at 400 degrees F for 20 - 25 minutes.

Yield: 12 servings

Calories: 106
Exchanges: *1*   *Bread*

Cholesterol: *<1 Mg*
SF: *0 Gm*
Fat: *<1 Gm*
Sodium: *154 Mg*
Dietary Fiber: *1 Gm*

PECAN MUFFINS

2 cups basic muffin mix
¼ cup egg substitute
½ cup skim milk
⅓ cup applesauce, unsweetened
½ cup chopped pecans

Mix all ingredients, except pecans. Do not overbeat. Fold in pecans. Fill muffin tins prepared with vegetable cooking spray or paper liners ⅔ full. Bake at 400 degrees F for 20 - 25 minutes.

Yield: 12 servings

Calories: 133
Exchanges: *1*   *Bread*
           ½   *Fat*

Cholesterol: *<1 Mg*
SF: *<1 Gm*
Fat: *3 Gm*
Sodium: *151 Mg*
Dietary Fiber: *1 Gm*

BRAN MUFFINS

1¼ cups all purpose flour
1 tablespoon baking powder
½ table salt
½ cup sugar
1½ cups Bran Buds cereal
1¼ cups 1% milk
1 egg
⅓ cup sweetened applesauce

Stir together flour, baking powder, salt and sugar. Set aside. Measure cereal and milk into large mixing bowl. Stir to combine. Let stand 1 to 2 minutes, until cereal is softened. Add egg and applesauce. Beat well. Add flour mixture, stirring only until combined. Spray (2½") muffin tins with non-stick spray or use paper liners. Fill 12 muffin cups. Bake in 400 degree F oven for about 25 minutes or until lightly browned. Three cups of raisin bran may be substituted for Bran Buds. The total fiber content, however will decrease.

Yield: 12 servings

Calories: 132
Exchanges: 1½ Bread

Cholesterol: 23 Mg
SF: <1 Gm
Fat: 1   Gm
Sodium: 239 Mg
Dietary Fiber: 3   Gm

OAT MUFFINS

½ **cup One Minute oatmeal, uncooked**
1 **cup bread flour**
1 **teaspoon baking powder**
½ **cup sugar**
½ **teaspoon salt**
¼ **cup egg substitute**
½ **cup skim milk**
⅓ **cup applesauce, unsweetened**

Mix dry ingredients. Gradually add remaining ingredients. Do not overbeat. Spoon into muffin tins prepared with vegetable cooking spray or paper liners ⅔ full. Bake at 400 degrees F for 20 - 25 minutes.

Yield: 12 muffins

Calories: 96
Exchanges: 1   Bread

Cholesterol: <1 Mg
SF: 0   Gm
Fat: <1 Gm
Sodium: 151 Mg
Dietary Fiber: 1   Gm

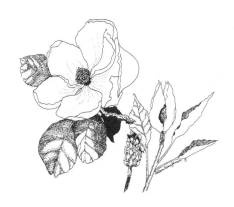

BANANA NUT BREAD

1½ cups all purpose flour
½ cup sugar
2½ teaspoons baking powder
½ teaspoon salt
½ teaspoon baking soda
1 cup Wheat Chex cereal
½ cup chopped pecans
1 egg
¼ cup sweetened applesauce
2 tablespoons water
1½ cups mashed bananas
1 teaspoon vanilla extract
    vegetable cooking spray

Spray 2 loaf pans (5" x 9") with cooking spray. Stir together flour, sugar, baking powder, salt, baking soda, cereal and nuts. Combine egg, applesauce, water, mashed banana and vanilla. Add all at once to dry ingredients. Stir slightly to moisten. Pour or spread in loaf pans. Bake 50 to 55 minutes at 350 degrees F or until loaves test done. Stick with clean toothpick. If the pick comes out clean, bread is done.

Yield: 36 (½" thick slice) servings

Calories: 95
Exchanges: *1*   *Bread*
              ½   *Fat*

Cholesterol: *15 Mg*
SF: *<1 Gm*
Fat: *3 Gm*
Sodium: *152 Mg*
Dietary Fiber: *1 Gm*

CINNAMON ROLLS

4 cups white bread flour
1 package active dry yeast
1½ teaspoons salt
1¼ cups water
½ cup sugar
1 teaspoon vanilla
½ teaspoon cinnamon
2 cups powdered sugar
2 tablespoons margarine

ROLLS:

Preheat oven to 375 degrees F. Combine yeast and warm water. Set aside. Place flour and salt in food processor. Turn processor on. While machine is running gradually add liquid. When dough works into a ball. Allow machine to knead dough (about 10 rounds in the machine.) Put dough into a bowl that has been sprayed with cooking spray. Let dough rise about an hour at room temperature. You may also put in an airtight container and place in the refrigerator overnight. (Be sure to leave room for dough to rise in the container). Roll dough out into a rectangle. Spread dough with sugar, cinnamon and vanilla. Roll up jelly roll style. Slice into 24 slices. Place into a 13" x 9" pan that has been sprayed with cooking spray. Place in oven. Bake 10 to 12 minutes.

ICING:

Melt margarine in microwave. Add powdered sugar and vanilla. Drizzle this mixture over hot rolls.

Yield: 24 servings

Calories: 139
Exchanges: Not acceptable for diabetics.

Cholesterol: *0* *Mg*
SF: *<1 Gm*
Fat: *1* *Gm*
Sodium: *155 Mg*
Dietary Fiber: 1 *Gm*

MAPLE CRUMB COFFEE CAKE

TOPPING:

⅓ cup brown sugar, packed
3 tablespoons all purpose flour
1 teaspoon cinnamon
½ ounce margarine
1 teaspoon maple flavoring

BATTER:

2 cups all purpose flour
2¼ teaspoons baking powder
¾ cup sugar
¾ teaspoon salt
2 medium eggs
½ cup applesauce
½ cup non fat skim milk
vegetable cooking spray

TOPPING:

Combine brown sugar, flour and cinnamon in small mixing bowl or food processor. Blend margarine and maple flavoring thoroughly into flour mixture. Set aside.

BATTER:

Sift together flour, baking powder, sugar and salt into mixing bowl. Combine beaten eggs, milk and applesauce, stirring into the dry ingredients until barely blended. Pour batter into 9" square pan that has been sprayed with cooking spray. Pour or spoon topping over batter. Bake at 400 degrees F for 30 minutes, until done.

Yield: 9 (3" square) servings

Calories: 254
Exchanges: Not acceptable for diabetics.

Cholesterol: *58 Mg*
SF: *1 Gm*
Fat: *3 Gm*
Sodium: *282 Mg*
Dietary Fiber: 1 Gm

EASY DINNER ROLLS

1	package yeast
1	cup water
2	tablespoons sugar
1	teaspoon salt
¼	cup egg substitute
2	tablespoons vegetable oil
1¼	cups all purpose flour

Dissolve yeast in warm water in large mixer bowl. Add sugar, salt, egg substitute, oil and 1 cup flour. Beat until smooth. Stir in remaining flour. Continue beating until smooth. Scrape batter from side of bowl. Cover. Let rise in warm place until double in size. Punch down batter and spoon into muffin tins prepared with cooking spray. Let rise until double. Heat oven to 400 degrees F. Bake about 15 minutes. Spray with butter flavored cooking spray when removed from oven, if desired.

Yield: 16

Calories: 88
Exchanges: *1*   *Bread*

Cholesterol: *0*   *Mg*
SF: *0*   *Gm*
Fat: *2*   *Gm*
Sodium: *139 Mg*
Dietary Fiber: *<1 Gm*

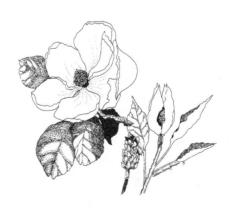

DELICIOUS YEAST ROLLS

1¼ cups skim evaporated milk
2 tablespoons honey
1¼ teaspoons salt
1 package yeast
¼ cup warm (105 - 110 degrees F) water
3 cups white bread flour
vegetable cooking spray
⅓ cup wheat germ

Combine first 4 ingredients in bowl. Mix and cool to lukewarm temperature. Dissolve yeast in warm water. Stir into milk mixture. Gradually add flour and wheat germ, mixing well after each addition, until a stiff dough is formed. Turn dough onto lightly floured board. Knead until dough is smooth and elastic. Place dough in bowl sprayed with cooking spray. Spray top of dough well with cooking spray. Cover with damp towel. Let rest in a warm place until double in size. Punch down and let sit 10 minutes. Shape into 24 rolls. Place on baking pan prepared with cooking spray. Spray top of rolls with cooking spray. Cover. Let rise until almost double in size. Bake in a 400 degree F oven until done, about 15 - 20 minutes.

Yield: 24 servings

Calories: 89
Exchanges: *1*   *Bread*

Cholesterol: *1*   *Mg*
SF: *<1*   *Gm*
Fat: *1*   *Gm*
Sodium: *137* *Mg*
Dietary Fiber: *1*   *Gm*

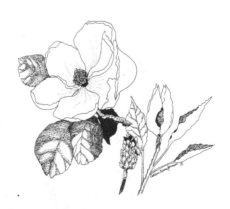

DESSERTS

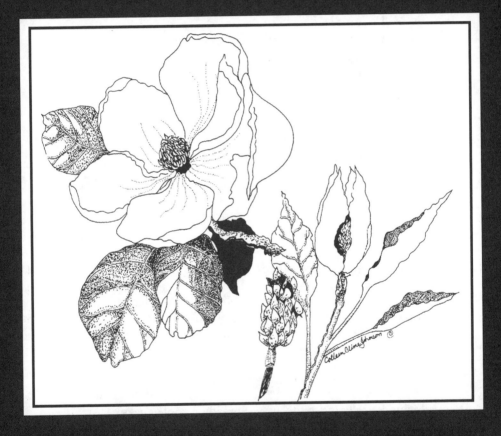

Colleen Cline Johnson ©

FRESH APPLE CAKE

CAKE:

1½ cups canned sweetened applesauce
2 cups sugar
2 cups all purpose flour
2 teaspoons ground cinnamon
1 teaspoon salt
2 teaspoons baking soda
1 cup diced raw apples
1 tablespoon vanilla extract
1 cup egg substitute
    vegetable cooking spray

ICING:

3 ounces light cream cheese
1½ cups powdered sugar
1 teaspoon vanilla
1 teaspoon evaporated skim milk

CAKE:

Preheat oven to 375 degrees F. Peel and chop apples. Set aside. Cream applesauce and sugar in food processor or mixer until well blended. About 4 minutes on high. Add egg substitute. Beat well. Sift dry ingredients. Stir in apples. Add flour mixture and vanilla. Mix well. Pour batter into a 13" x 9" pan that has been sprayed with vegetable cooking spray. Bake for 30 - 35 minutes or until an inserted toothpick comes out clean. Remove cake from oven and let cool.

ICING:

Beat all icing ingredients until fluffy. Spread on cooled cake.

Yield: 12 servings

Calories: 312
Exchanges: Not acceptable for diabetics.

Cholesterol: 3 *Mg*
SF: <1 *Gm*
Fat: 2 *Gm*
Sodium: 460 *Mg*
Dietary Fiber: 1 *Gm*

APPLE SPICE CAKE

2¾ cups all purpose flour
1¼ cups sugar
2½ teaspoons baking soda
1¼ teaspoons baking powder
1 teaspoon ground cinnamon
1 teaspoon salt
1¾ cups unsweetened canned applesauce
1¼ cups plain nonfat yogurt
½ cup substitute egg product
⅓ cup corn oil
1 cup seedless raisins
3 tablespoons brown sugar packed
1 teaspoon pure vanilla
1½ cups plain non fat yogurt

CAKE:

In a large bowl, combine flour, sugar, baking soda, baking powder, cinnamon, and salt. Mix well. Add applesauce, 1¼ cups of yogurt, egg substitute, and oil. Blend well using a spoon. Stir in raisins. Pour into Bundt pan or 13" x 9" pan prepared with non-stick vegetable spray. Bake at 325 degrees F for 50 - 60 minutes or until toothpick comes out clean. Cool 15 minutes. Loosen cake from sides of pan with knife and invert onto a plate. Cover loosely with foil. Cool completely.

GLAZE:

Mix 1½ cups of non fat plain yogurt, 3 tablespoons brown sugar and 1 teaspoon vanilla until smooth.

Yield: 24 servings

Calories: 200
Exchanges: 2 *Bread*
½ *Fat*

Cholesterol: 11 *Mg*
SF: <1 *Gm*
Fat: 3 *Gm*
Sodium: 255 *Mg*
Dietary Fiber: 1 *Gm*

BLUEBERRY BATTER CAKE

2   cups blueberries, frozen or fresh
3   tablespoons lemon juice
1   cup all purpose flour
1½ cups sugar
1   teaspoon baking powder
2   tablespoons diet margarine
½   cup skim milk
2   tablespoons cornstarch
1   cup boiling water
   vegetable cooking spray

Prepare a 11" x 7" pan with non-stick vegetable spray. Place blueberries in pan. Sprinkle lemon juice over blueberries. Mix flour, 1 cup sugar, baking powder, margarine and milk well. Pour over the blueberries. Mix ½ cup sugar and 2 teaspoons cornstarch and pour over batter. Pour 1 cup boiling water over this. Bake at 350 degrees F until brown and done.

Yield: 8 servings

Calories: 274
Exchanges: Not acceptable for diabetics.

Cholesterol: *<1 Mg*
SF: *<1 Gm*
Fat: *2 Gm*
Sodium: *45 Mg*
Dietary Fiber: *2 Gm*

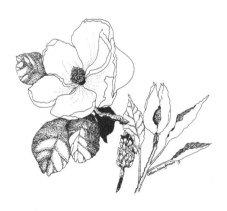

CHOCOLATE SNACK CAKE

	vegetable cooking spray
1¼	cups all purpose flour
½	cup cocoa
¼	cup cornstarch
1	teaspoon baking powder
½	teaspoon baking soda
½	teaspoon salt
1¼	cups brown sugar, packed
1	cup water
3	egg whites
½	cup corn syrup

Preheat oven to 350 degrees F. Spray a 9 x 9" baking pan with cooking spray. In a large bowl, combine flour, cocoa cornstarch, baking powder, baking soda and salt. In medium bowl with wire whisk or fork. Stir sugar and water for 1 minute. Add egg whites and corn syrup. Stir until blended. Gradually stir into dry ingredients until smooth. Pour into pan. Bake 35 minutes or until toothpick inserted in center comes out clean. Cool. If desired sprinkle with confectioners sugar.

Yield: 16 servings

Calories: 150
Exchanges: Not acceptable for diabetics.

Cholesterol:	*0*	*Mg*
SF:	*0*	*Gm*
Fat:	*<1*	*Gm*
Sodium:	*139*	*Mg*
Dietary Fiber:	*<1*	*Gm*

CHIFFON CAKE WITH KAHLUA FROSTING

CAKE:

1	cup cake flour
1	cup sugar
1½	teaspoons baking powder
¼	teaspoon salt
⅓	cup unsweetened applesauce
4	eggs
¼	cup water
1	teaspoon vanilla extract
½	teaspoon cream of tartar

ICING:

2	tablespoons powdered sugar
2	tablespoons Kahlua
1	teaspoon vanilla extract
1	teaspoon instant coffee powder
1	teaspoon water
8	ounce carton of light Cool Whip

CAKE:

Sift together flour, ½ cup sugar, baking powder and salt in a mixing bowl. Make a well in the center. Add applesauce, egg yolks, water and vanilla. Beat with an electric beater at high speed for about 5 minutes or until satiny. (Set aside) Beat egg whites (at room temperature) and cream of tartar in a large mixing bowl until soft peaks form. Add remaining ½ cup of sugar, one table-spoon full at a time and beat until stiff peaks form. Pour egg yolk mixture in a thin, steady stream over the entire surface of egg whites. Gently fold into mixture. Pour batter into an ungreased 10" tube pan. Spread evenly with a spatula. Bake at 325 degrees F for 1 hour until cake springs back when lightly touched. Invert pan. Cook 40 minutes. Loosen cake from sides using a narrow metal spatula. Remove from pan.

(Continued on next page)

(Chiffon Cake with Kahlua Frosting, continued)

ICING:

Combine 2 tablespoons Kahlua, 1 teaspoon instant coffee powder and 1 teaspoon water. Stir until smooth. Add powdered sugar and 1 teaspoon vanilla to Kahlua mixture. Fold Kahlua mixture into Cool Whip. This cake will need to be refrigerated.

Yield: 12 servings

Calories: 185
Exchanges: Not acceptable for diabetics.

Cholesterol:	*71*	*Mg*
SF:	*1*	*Gm*
Fat:	*1*	*Gm*
Sodium:	*83*	*Mg*
Dietary Fiber:	*<1*	*Gm*

QUICK DUMP CAKE

- **1 can apple pie filling**
- **1 large can pineapple bits, water packed**
- **1 box light yellow cake mix**
- **1 cup liquid Butter Buds**

Dump pie filling in a shallow 2 quart casserole dish. Add pineapple. Sprinkle dry cake mix over fruit. Pour butter substitute on top. Bake at 350 degrees F for 35 - 40 minutes.

Serving suggestion: May top with a scoop of fat free yogurt or fat free ice cream while warm.

Yield: 16 servings

Calories: 132
Exchanges: Not acceptable for diabetics.

Cholesterol:	*17*	*Mg*
SF:	*<1*	*Gm*
Fat:	*2*	*Gm*
Sodium:	*336*	*Mg*
Dietary Fiber:	*1*	*Gm*

PINEAPPLE UPSIDE DOWN CAKE

	vegetable cooking spray
¼	cup brown sugar, packed
2	tablespoons corn syrup
2	tablespoons lemon juice
8	ounces sliced pineapple, water packed
1	cup all purpose flour
¼	cup cornstarch
1½	teaspoons baking powder
½	teaspoon salt
1	cup sugar
⅔	cup skim milk
2	egg whites
⅓	cup corn syrup
1	teaspoon vanilla
7	maraschino cherries

Preheat oven to 350 degrees F. Spray a 9" round cake pan with cooking spray. Add brown sugar, corn syrup and lemon. Stir to combine. Place pan in oven 3 minutes. Remove. Arrange pineapple rings and cherries in pan. Set aside. In a large bowl, combine flour, cornstarch, baking powder and salt. In a medium bowl mix sugar and milk and stir with a wire whisk or a fork for 1 minute. Add egg whites, corn syrup and vanilla. Stir until blended. Gradually stir into flour mixture until smooth. Spoon batter over pineapple. Bake for 35 - 40 minutes or until toothpick inserted in center comes out clean. Immediately loosen cake from pan. Invert onto serving plate.

Yield: 12 servings

Calories: 187
Exchanges: Not acceptable for diabetics.

Cholesterol:	*<1 Mg*
SF:	*0 Gm*
Fat:	*<1 Gm*
Sodium:	*116 Mg*
Dietary Fiber:	*1 Gm*

SPICED SWEET POTATO CAKE

CAKE:

2 cups sugar
1 cup egg substitute
1 cup unsweetened applesauce
2 cups boiled, mashed sweet potatoes
2 cups all purpose flour
1 teaspoon ground cinnamon
½ teaspoon salt
2 teaspoons baking powder
1 teaspoon baking soda
vegetable cooking spray

Cream sugar, egg substitute and apple sauce until light. (This does well in food processor). Add mashed sweet potatoes. Mix until smooth. Stir in dry ingredients. Pour batter into two 9" cake pans that have been sprayed with vegetable cooking spray. Bake at 350 degrees F for 40 minutes. While cake is baking, make 7 Minute Icing.

7 MINUTE ICING:

1½ cups sugar
2 egg whites
⅓ cup water
2 teaspoons corn syrup
dash of salt
1 teaspoon vanilla

In the top of a double boiler combine sugar, egg whites, ⅓ cup water, 1 teaspoons light corn syrup and a dash of salt. Beat 1 minute with an electric mixer until well combined. Place pot over boiling water. Add vanilla and beat until frosting is of spreading consistency.

Yield: 16 servings

Calories: 287
Exchanges: Not acceptable for diabetics.

Cholesterol: *0*   *Mg*
SF: *0*   *Gm*
Fat: *<1* *Gm*
Sodium: *199* *Mg*
Dietary Fiber: *2*   *Gm*

SOUTHERN BLACKBERRY COBBLER

5	**cups fresh blackberries or frozen without sugar**
¾	**cup white sugar**
2	**cups all purpose flour**
2	**teaspoons all purpose flour**
½	**teaspoon baking powder**
½	**teaspoon baking soda**
½	**cup plain nonfat yogurt**
2	**tablespoons light margarine**
1	**teaspoon vanilla extract**
2	**egg whites**
	vegetable cooking spray

Combine blackberries, sugar and 2 tablespoons flour. Spoon this mixture into an 11" x 7" x 2" baking pan coated with non-stick vegetable spray. Set aside. Combine yogurt and remaining ingredients, add to dry ingredients, stirring just until mixture is moistened. Drop dough by tablespoons onto blackberry mixture. Bake at 400 degrees F for 30 minutes or until filling is bubbly and crust is brown. Serve warm.

Yield: 8 servings

Calories: 210
Exchanges: Not acceptable for diabetics.

Cholesterol:	*<1 Mg*
SF:	*<1 Gm*
Fat:	*2 Gm*
Sodium:	*131 Mg*
Dietary Fiber:	*6 Gm*

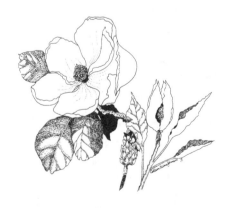

CHERRY COBBLER WITH CRUMB TOPPING

1 can cherry pie filling
2 tablespoons light margarine
½ cup raw one minute oatmeal
4 tablespoons all purpose flour
½ cup sugar
2 tablespoons chopped pecans
butter flavored vegetable spray

Spray a 2 quart casserole with cooking spray. Open can of cherry pie filling. Pour into casserole. Mix light margarine, oatmeal, flour, sugar and pecans. Crumble over cherry pie filling. Bake at 350 degrees F for 20 to 25 minutes.

Yield: 8 servings

Calories: 173
Exchanges: Not acceptable for diabetics.

Cholesterol: *0*   *Mg*
SF: *<1*   *Gm*
Fat: *3*   *Gm*
Sodium: *24*   *Mg*
Dietary Fiber: *1*   *Gm*

QUICK AND EASY PEACH COBBLER

1 can (20 ounces) peach halves in light syrup
1 cup sugar
1 cup low fat Pioneer biscuit mix
butter flavored cooking spray

Spray a 3 quart casserole with butter flavored cooking spray. Combine all ingredients. Mix well. Spoon into casserole. Bake at 350 degrees F for 35 - 40 minutes or until golden brown.

Yield: 8 servings

Calories: 241
Exchanges: Not acceptable for diabetics.

Cholesterol: *0*   *Mg*
SF: *0*   *Gm*
Fat: *1*   *Gm*
Sodium: *487*   *Mg*
Dietary Fiber: *1*   *Gm*

PEACH COBBLER

COBBLER:

½ cup sugar
2 tablespoons cornstarch
¾ cup water
1 tablespoon dry butter substitute granules
¼ teaspoon cinnamon
3 cups frozen or fresh sliced peaches

Combine cornstarch and a small amount of water. Stir Well. Add remaining water. Continue to stir well. Place cornstarch mixture, butter substitute, cinnamon, sugar and peaches in saucepan. Cook on medium heat until mixture is thickened. Stir occasionally. Pour cobbler mixture into a square casserole dish prepared with cooking spray.

CRUST:

½ cup flour
⅓ cup sugar
⅓ cup skim evaporated milk
½ teaspoon baking powder
    dash of salt
½ teaspoon vanilla
1 tablespoon diet margarine

Mix all crust ingredients well to make a batter. Pour crust batter on top of cobbler mixture. Bake at 350 degrees F for 35 - 40 minutes or until golden brown.

Yield: 8 servings

Calories: 140
Exchanges: Not acceptable for diabetics.

Cholesterol: *0*   *Mg*
SF: *<1*   *Gm*
Fat: *<1*   *Gm*
Sodium: *72*   *Mg*
Dietary Fiber: *1*   *Gm*

LIGHT CHOCOLATE BROWNIES

6 tablespoons light margarine
1 cup sugar
1 teaspoon vanilla
½ cup cocoa
½ cup egg substitute
½ cup all purpose flour
¼ cup chopped pecans
2 tablespoons powdered sugar
   vegetable cooking spray

Preheat oven to 350 degrees F. Lightly spray an 8" square pan with non-stick cooking spray. In medium saucepan over low heat, melt margarine. Add sugar. Stir until well blended. Remove from heat. Stir in cocoa and vanilla. Add egg substitute. Stir to blend. Stir in flour and pecans. Pour batter into 8" cake pan. Bake 25 minutes. Cool in pan on wire rack. Sprinkle with powdered sugar. Cut into 16 squares.

Yield: 16 servings

Calories: 114
Exchanges: Not acceptable for diabetics.

Cholesterol: *0*   *Mg*
SF: *<1*   *Gm*
Fat: *4*   *Gm*
Sodium: *32*   *Mg*
Dietary Fiber: *<1*   *Gm*

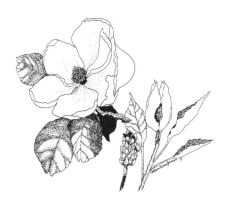

OLD FASHIONED LEMON SQUARES

1 cup all purpose flour
⅓ cup white powdered sugar, unsifted
¼ cup corn oil margarine
   butter flavored cooking spray
1 cup sugar
2 tablespoons all purpose flour
½ teaspoon baking powder
¼ teaspoon salt
3 egg whites
1 egg
7 tablespoons lemon juice
¼ teaspoon butter extract
2 tablespoons white powdered sugar, sifted

CRUST:

Combine 1 cup flour and ⅓ cup powdered sugar in a bowl. Cut in margarine with a pastry blender until resembles course meal. Press this into bottom of an 11" x 7" x 2" baking dish coated with cooking spray. Bake at 350 degrees F for 20 minutes or until lightly browned.

TOPPING:

Combine sugar and next 5 ingredients in a bowl, stirring well. Stir in lemon juice and butter extract. Pour mixture over crust. Bake at 350 degrees F for 20 minutes. Cool completely. Sift 2 tablespoons sifted powdered sugar over squares. Cut in 2" squares.

Yield: 24 servings

Calories: 87 per square
Exchanges: Not acceptable for diabetics.

Cholesterol:	*11*	*Mg*
SF:	*<1*	*Gm*
Fat:	*2*	*Gm*
Sodium	*60*	*Mg*
Dietary Fiber:	*<1*	*Gm*

LOW FAT EASY BAKE COOKIES

1 box light yellow cake mix
¼ cup egg substitute
¼ cup canned unsweetened applesauce
¼ cup water
   vegetable cooking spray

Mix all ingredients until well blended by hand. Lightly spray cookie sheet with vegetable cooking spray. Drop by rounded teaspoons onto cookie sheet. Bake at 350 degrees F until lightly brown.

Yield: 60 cookies (5 dozen)

Calories: 36
Exchanges: Not acceptable for diabetics.

Cholesterol:	*0*	*Mg*
SF:	*<1*	*Gm*
Fat:	*1*	*Gm*
Sodium:	*59*	*Mg*
Dietary Fiber:	*<1*	*Gm*

FLOWER POT DESSERT

12 ounces light whipped topping
 8 Snackwell chocolate wafer cookies, crushed
 1 ounce green sprinkles
 8 cups fat free ice cream or frozen yogurt

Combine fat free ice cream or yogurt, 12 ounces light whipped topping and crushed cookies. To close the holes , place 1 small piece of aluminum foil in the bottom of 10, 2½" clay flower pots. Spoon ice cream mixture into flower pot. Sprinkle top of mixture with green sprinkles. Cut a drinking straw in half and insert 1 piece in the center of mixture. Freeze until serving time. Place a live flower in the straw. (Green sprinkles are easily found in the grocery store with cake decorating items).

Yield: 10 servings

Calories: 282
Exchanges: Not acceptable for diabetics.

Cholesterol:	*1*	*Mg*
SF:	*0*	*Gm*
Fat:	*5*	*Gm*
Sodium:	*170*	*Mg*
Dietary Fiber:	*3*	*Gm*

CHERRY GELATIN DELIGHT

2 small boxes of cherry gelatin
1 cup boiling water
¾ cup cold water
1 20 ounce can crushed pineapple
1 20 ounce can cherry pie filling
8 ounces fat free cream cheese
8 ounces fat free sour cream
½ cup white powdered sugar
1 teaspoon vanilla

FILLING:

Dissolve gelatin with 2 cups of boiling water and add ¾ cup cold water. Blend in pineapple in its own juice, along with the cherry pie filling. Pour into a 9" x 13" dish and refrigerate until completely set.

TOPPING:

Beat 8 ounces of fat free cream cheese, vanilla, fat free sour cream and sugar. Spread on top of gelatin mixture. Decorate with several cherries from the pie filling if desired. This may be made one or two days ahead.

Yield: 12 servings

Calories: 218
Exchanges: Not acceptable for diabetics.

Cholesterol: *3*   *Mg*
SF: *0*   *Gm*
Fat: *1*   *Gm*
Sodium: *165 Mg*
Dietary Fiber: *<1 Gm*

ORANGE CHARLOTTE

1 **package dry gelatin**
¾ **cup water**
1 **cup sugar**
1 **cup orange juice**
2 **tablespoons lemon juice**
8 **tablespoons light Cool Whip**

In a mixing bowl, dissolve gelatin in ¼ cup cold water. Let stand 5 minutes. Add ½ cup boiling water, sugar, orange juice and lemon juice. Stir until sugar is dissolved. Let set in refrigerator until it has the consistency of egg whites. It is important that the mixture sets long enough to be softly set, but not too firm. If not it will settle on the bottom. Beat egg whites until stiff enough to hold peaks. Fold egg whites into gelatin mixture until blended. Chill several hours. Top with light Cool Whip.

Frozen orange juice concentrate may be used. Dilute with only ⅔ the amount of water listed on the container.

Yield: 4 servings

Calories: 121
Exchanges: Not acceptable for diabetics.

Cholesterol: *<1 Mg*
SF: *<1 Gm*
Fat: *<1 Gm*
Sodium: *5 Mg*
Dietary Fiber: *0 Gm*

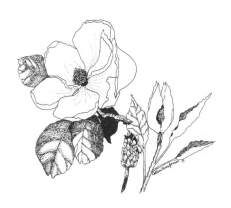

STRAWBERRY DREAM

DESSERT:

1 package unflavored gelatin
¼ cup water
1 package Healthy Choice strawberry fat free cream cheese
½ cup sugar
½ teaspoon vanilla
  dash salt
1 cup skim milk
8 tablespoons light Cool Whip

Combine gelatin and water in a small saucepan. Cook over low heat. Stir until gelatin dissolves. Set aside. Combine cream cheese, sugar, vanilla and dash of salt. Beat until smooth and creamy. Gradually add milk and gelatin mixture to creamed mixture. Mix well. Fold in light Cool Whip in gelatin mixture. Pour into a 4-cup mold that has been sprayed with cooking spray. Chill until set. Unmold dessert onto a serving dish. Serve with strawberry sauce.

Yield: 8 servings

SAUCE:

10 ounces frozen strawberries, sliced
1 tablespoon cornstarch
1 ounce dry sherry
  vegetable cooking spray

Drain strawberries. Reserve juice. Put strawberries in food processor. Set pulp aside. Combine juice, cornstarch and sherry in a small saucepan. Mix well. Cook over low heat. Stir constantly until smooth and slightly thickened. Stir in strawberries. Cool.

Yield: 1 cup

Calories: 141
Exchanges: Not acceptable for diabetics.

Cholesterol: *4*   *Mg*
SF: *0*   *Gm*
Fat: *1*   *Gm*
Sodium: *257 Mg*
Dietary Fiber: *1*   *Gm*

DEEP DISH STRAWBERRY PIE

1   cup cake flour
1   cup sugar
1   teaspoon baking powder
¼   cup light margarine
1   cup plus 2 tablespoons water
    vegetable cooking spray
4   cups strawberries, sliced
4   ounces light whipped topping

Combine flour, 2 tablespoons sugar and margarine in bowl. Cut in margarine with a pastry blender in fine pieces resembling coarse meal. Sprinkle with 2 tablespoons water and stir until ingredients are moistened. Shape dough into a ball. Place dough between 2 sheets of plastic wrap and roll into a 12" circle. Remove top sheet of wrap and invert dough on to 10" deep dish pie plate that has been prepared with cooking spray. Crimp edges of crust if desired. Bake crust in a 375 degree F oven until brown. Mix cornstarch with water. Add strawberries and remaining sugar to boiler. Cook over medium heat until thickened and bubbly. Stir constantly. Let cook 10 minutes. Pour strawberry mixture into cooled pie shell and top with light whipped topping.

Yield: 10 servings

Calories: 184
Exchanges: Not acceptable for diabetics.

Cholesterol: *<1 Mg*
SF: *<1 Gm*
Fat: *4 Gm*
Sodium: *59 Mg*
Dietary Fiber: *<1 Gm*

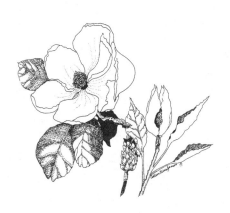

BANANA PUDDING

3 bananas
1 teaspoon cornstarch
2 cups canned skim evaporated milk
¾ cup egg beaters
½ cup plus 2 tablespoons sugar
36 vanilla wafers

CRUST:

In a deep baking dish, place 12 vanilla wafers, standing some on the edge of the bowl. Place one sliced banana over the wafers. Repeat this step until you have 2 more layers.

CUSTARD:

Beat ¾ cup of eggbeaters slightly. Add ½ cup of sugar and 1 tablespoon of cornstarch to eggbeaters. Add 2 cups of scalded skim evaporated milk and cook over a double boiler until the custard thickens, stirring constantly. Pour custard over the bananas and wafers.

TOPPING:

Beat 3 eggs whites with 4 tablespoons of sugar until stiff. Spread this over the contents of the dish and bake in a 325 degree F oven for 15 - 20 minutes.

Yield: 8 (1 cup) servings

Calories: 231
Exchanges: Not acceptable for diabetics.

Cholesterol:	*2*	*Mg*
SF:	*0*	*Gm*
Fat:	*<1*	*Gm*
Sodium:	*278*	*Mg*
Dietary Fiber:	*<1*	*Gm*

QUICK BANANA PUDDING

2   small boxes of instant vanilla pudding
3   cups skim milk
1   cup fat free sour cream
1   cup light Cool Whip
6   sliced bananas
24 vanilla wafers

TO MAKE IT LIGHT:

2   small boxes of sugar free instant vanilla pudding
    all other ingredients remain the same

With an electric mixer, beat on low the milk and pudding until creamy. Blend in fat free sour cream and Cool Whip until smooth. Layer pudding mix with bananas and vanilla wafers.

Yield: 8 servings

Calories: 281 (with sugar) - 202 (light)
Exchanges: (light): ½ Bread
                 1½ Fruit
                 ½ Milk

Cholesterol: *1*   *Mg*
SF: *1*   *Gm*
Fat: *2*   *Gm*
Sodium: *442 Mg*
Dietary Fiber: *2*   *Gm*

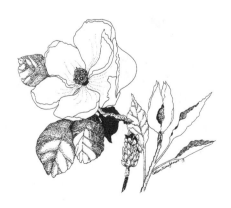

RICE PUDDING

2 cups long grain rice, cooked
½ cup sugar
½ cup egg substitute
1⅕ cups evaporated skim milk
1 teaspoon vanilla
¼ teaspoon ground nutmeg
½ cup seedless raisins

Mix cooked rice and raisins in a 1 quart casserole. Set aside. In a mixing bowl, blend together remaining ingredients. Pour over rice and raisins. Place casserole in a pan of hot water. Bake at 350 degrees F for 1 hour. Cool and serve.

Yield: 8 servings

Calories: 173
Exchanges: Not acceptable for diabetics.

Cholesterol: 2 *Mg*
SF: <1 *Gm*
Fat: <1 *Gm*
Sodium: 77 *Mg*
Dietary Fiber: <1 *Gm*

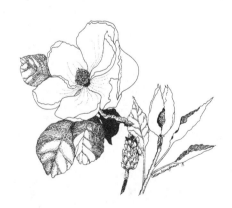

THE GOOD

AND THE

BAD

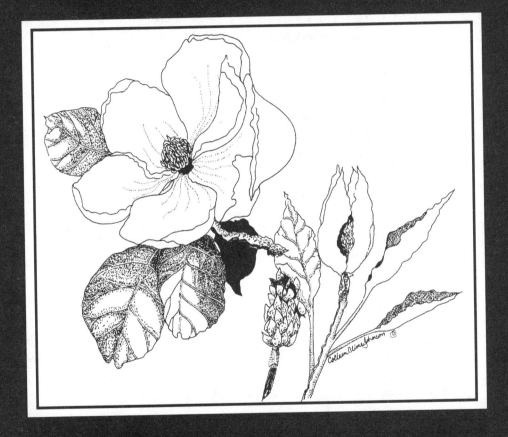

CARROT CAKE - LIGHT RECIPE

CAKE:

1½ cups applesauce
2 cups sugar
2 cups all purpose flour
2 eggs
2 teaspoons baking soda
2 teaspoons cinnamon
1 teaspoon salt
3 cups shredded carrots

ICING:

4 ounces cream cheese
3½ cups confectioners sugar
2 teaspoons vanilla
2 tablespoons skim milk

CAKE:

Beat eggs, sugar and applesauce. Mix well. Mix and add dry ingredients to mixture. Add shredded carrots. Mix well and pour into 13" x 9" cake pan. Bake at 350 degrees F for 40 minutes. Cool on cake rack. Ice with cream cheese icing.

ICING:

Cream powdered sugar and cream cheese. Add vanilla and skim milk. Mix well. Spread on cool cake.

Yield: 12 servings

Calories: 195
Exchanges: Not acceptable for diabetics.

Cholesterol: *48 Mg*
SF: *1 Gm*
Fat: *3 Gm*
Sodium: *231 Mg*
Dietary Fiber: *1 Gm*

CARROT CAKE - TRADITIONAL RECIPE

CAKE:

1½	cups vegetable oil
2	cups sugar
2	cups all purpose flour
2	eggs
2	teaspoons baking soda
2	teaspoons cinnamon
1	teaspoon salt
3	cups shredded carrots
½	cup chopped pecans

ICING:

1	package (8 ounces) cream cheese
3½	cups sugar
8	tablespoons butter
2	teaspoons vanilla
1	cup shredded coconut
½	cup chopped pecans

CAKE:

Beat eggs, add sugar and oil gradually. Mix well. Mix and add dry ingredients to mixture. Add shredded carrots and ½ cup pecans. Bake in 3 9" cake pans at 350 degrees F for 40 minutes. Cool on cake rack. Ice with cream cheese icing.

ICING:

Cream butter and cream cheese. Add powdered sugar, coconut, ½ cup pecans and vanilla. Mix well. Spread on cool cake.

Yield: 12 servings

Calories: 852
Exchanges: Not acceptable for diabetics.

Cholesterol:	*77*	*Mg*
SF:	*16*	*Gm*
Fat:	*52*	*Gm*
Sodium:	*573*	*Mg*
Dietary Fiber:	*3*	*Gm*

FAT FREE CHEESE CAKE

1½ cups sugar
3 tablespoons all purpose flour
2 tablespoons lemon juice
1¼ cups egg substitute
¾ cup graham cracker crumbs
1 tablespoon diet margarine
4 8 ounce packages fat free cream cheese
   vegetable cooking spray

Preheat oven to 450 degrees F. Blend graham cracker crumbs and margarine. Press into the bottom of a 10" spring form pan that has been sprayed with vegetable cooking spray. Cream sugar and cheese at low speed. You may use a food processor instead of a blender. When blended, add egg substitute, flour, and lemon juice. Mix well. Pour into spring form pan. Cook 12 minutes at 450 degrees F. Turn oven down (do not open oven door) to 300 degrees F and cook for 35 minutes. Turn oven off and allow cheese cake to stay in hot oven for 30 minutes more. Remove cheese cake and allow to cool completely. It is normal for the cheese cake to crack in some climates. This does not hurt the cake.

SUGAR FREE RECIPE:

72 packets Sweet and Low (use instead of sugar)
    all other ingredients remain the same

Follow the directions above substituting Sweet and Low for sugar. The diabetic exchanges below are for the sugar free recipe.

Yield: 16 servings

Calories: 175 (with sugar) - 122 (sugar free)
Exchanges: With sugar substitute:
        ½ Meat
        1 Bread

Cholesterol: *12 Mg*
SF: *<1 Gm*
Fat: *0   Gm*
Sodium: *487 Mg*
Dietary Fiber: *0   Gm*

NEW YORK CHEESE CAKE - TRADITIONAL

CRUST:

1   egg yolk
¾   cup margarine
¼   cup sugar
1¼ cups flour

Mix crust ingredients to form a dough. Chill 1 hour in refrigerator. Press dough in the bottom of a 10 inch springform pan. Cook 8 minutes in a preheated oven of 400 degrees F.

FILLING:

1   eggs
2½ tablespoons flour
5   packages (8 ounce each) cream cheese
¼   cup milk
1¾ cups sugar
2   tablespoons lemon juice

Cream the cheese and sugar at low speed. When blended, add eggs, flour, milk and lemon juice. Press remainingdough to sides of pan. Pour filling into crust. Cook 12 minutes in preheated 475 degree F oven, then turn down to 300 degrees for 30 minutes. Allow to cool completely. If cheesecake cracks while baking, that is okay.

Yield: 12 servings

Calories: 662
Exchanges: Not acceptable for diabetics.

Cholesterol: *226 Mg*
SF: *23 Gm*
Fat: *48 Gm*
Sodium: *485 Mg*
Dietary Fiber: 0 Gm

SNOW WHITE ICE CREAM - LIGHT RECIPE

3 cups sugar
2 tablespoons vanilla
1 gallon non fat buttermilk
2 cups half and half

Mix sugar and buttermilk in a large bowl, stirring until the sugar is completely dissolved. Add half and half and vanilla. Freeze in an electric freezer.

Yield: 16 (1 cup servings)

Calories: 276
Exchanges: Not acceptable for diabetics.

Cholesterol: *13   Mg*
SF: *2   Gm*
Fat: *3   Gm*
Sodium: *139 Mg*
Dietary Fiber: *0   Gm*

SNOW WHITE ICE CREAM - TRADITIONAL RECIPE

3 cups sugar
2 tablespoons vanilla
½ gallon buttermilk
1 cup heavy whipping cream

Mix sugar and buttermilk in a large bowl, stirring until the sugar is completely dissolved. Add whipping cream and vanilla. Freeze in an electric freezer.

Yield: 16 (1 cup) servings

Calories: 405
Exchanges: Not acceptable for diabetics.

Cholesterol: *86   Mg*
SF: *14   Gm*
Fat: *23   Gm*
Sodium: *151 Mg*
Dietary Fiber: *0   Gm*

LEMON MERINGUE PIE - LIGHT RECIPE

4	sheets phyllo dough
1½	cups water
6	teaspoons cornstarch
½	cup sugar
½	cup lemon juice
6	egg whites
1¼	teaspoons cream of tartar
2	tablespoons honey
1	cup egg substitute
	vegetable cooking spray

CRUST:

Prepare a 9" pie plate with non-stick cooking spray. Drape 1 sheet of phyllo dough across the plate. Press down into the plate, folding the edges toward the center. Mist with non-stick cooking spray. Repeat the layers with the remaining sheets and cooking spray. Bake at 375 degrees F until golden brown (5 to 7 minutes). Cool on a wire rack.

FILLING:

In a 2 quart saucepan, whisk the water and cornstarch until dissolved. Stir in sugar and lemon juice. Place over medium heat and cook, stirring constantly until mixture comes to a boil and begins to thicken and turn clear. Remove from heat and slowly whisk in egg substitute. Return to heat and cook until thickened. Set aside and cool to room temperature.

TOPPING:

Place egg whites in a dry, large bowl. Beat until foamy. Add cream of tartar and continue beating until soft peaks form. Drizzle in honey and beat until whites are stiff. Spoon filling into pie crust, making sure meringue is sealed to the outside edges. Cook at 400 degrees F until lightly browned.

Yield: 8 slices

Calories: 233
Exchanges: Not acceptable for diabetics.

Cholesterol:	*0*	*Mg*
SF:	*0*	*Gm*
Fat:	*<1*	*Gm*
Sodium:	*477*	*Mg*
Dietary Fiber:	*0*	*Gm*

LEMON MERINGUE PIE - TRADITIONAL RECIPE

1⅓   **cups sugar**
  3   **tablespoons cornstarch**
1½   **cups water**
  3   **eggs**
  ¼   **cup lemon juice**
  1   **tablespoon butter**
  1   **prepared pie crust**
  3   **egg whites**

FILLING:

Stir together 1 cup sugar and cornstarch in saucepan. Gradually stir in water until smooth. Stir in egg yolks. Stir constantly. Bring to a boil over medium heat and boil for 1 minute while stirring. Remove from heat. Stir in lemon juice and butter. Cool. Pour into pie shell.

MERINGUE:

Beat egg whites until foamy with mixer at high speed. Add ⅓ cup sugar, 1 tablespoon at a time. Beat after each addition. Beat until soft peaks form. Spread meringue around edge of filling, touching crust, then fill center. Bake in a 350 degree F oven 15 minutes until lightly browned. Cool.

Yield: 8 servings

Calories: 418
Exchanges: Not acceptable for diabetics.

Cholesterol: *99 Mg*
SF: *1   Gm*
Fat: *18 Gm*
Sodium: *246 Mg*
Dietary Fiber: *0   Gm*

PECAN PIE - LIGHT RECIPE

- 10 saltine crackers
- ¾ cup pecans
- 6 egg whites
- ¾ cup sugar
- ½ teaspoon vanilla

Finely grind pecans and crackers in a food processor with metal blade. Set aside. Beat egg whites at high speed with and electric mixer until foamy. Gradually add sugar. Beat until stiff peaks form. Fold in cracker mixture and vanilla extract. Spoon into a 9" pie plate prepared with cooking spray. Bake at 375 degrees F for 20 minutes or until browned. Serve with lite whipped topping or non fat frozen yogurt.

Yield: 8 servings

Calories: 169
Exchanges: Not acceptable for diabetics.

Cholesterol:	*<1*	*Mg*
SF:	*<1*	*Gm*
Fat:	*7*	*Gm*
Sodium:	*86*	*Mg*
Dietary Fiber:	*1*	*Gm*

PECAN PIE - TRADITIONAL RECIPE

- 3 eggs
- 1 cup light corn syrup
- ½ cup sugar
- ½ cup butter
- ¼ teaspoon salt
- 2 cups pecans, ground
- 1 pie crust

Put pie shell in a 350 degree F oven for 5 minutes. Mix all ingredients well. Pour mixture into pie shell. Return to the oven and bake for an additional 25 - 35 minutes at 350 degrees F.

Yield: 8 servings

Calories: 718
Exchanges: Not acceptable for diabetics.

Cholesterol:	*126*	*Mg*
SF:	*9*	*Gm*
Fat:	*47*	*Gm*
Sodium:	*446*	*Mg*
Dietary Fiber:	*2*	*Gm*

CHICKEN AND DRESSING - LIGHT RECIPE

CORNBREAD:

2   cups cornmeal
¾   cup all purpose flour
2½ teaspoons baking powder
¾   teaspoon baking soda
2   teaspoons sugar
2¼ cups low fat buttermilk
¾   cup egg substitute
    vegetable cooking spray

Preheat oven to 450 degrees F. Combine cornmeal, flour, baking powder, soda and sugar in bowl. Combine buttermilk and egg substitute. Add to dry ingredients, stirring just until moistened. Prepare 10" cast iron skillet with nonstick vegetable spray. Pour batter into skillet and bake 25 - 30 minutes or until golden brown. Let cool. Crumble cornbread into fine pieces.

DRESSING:

1   cup diced celery
½   cup chopped onion
2   16 ounce cans fat free chicken broth
½   teaspoon salt
    dash of black pepper
½   pound of skinless chicken breasts
2   tablespoons dry butter substitute
½   cup egg substitute

Cook celery and onion in non-stick skillet with cooking spray until tender. Transfer to large bowl. Mix in remaining ingredients. Spoon into 13" x 9" x 2" baking dish. Bake at 400 degrees F for 40 minutes or until brown.

Yield: 8 servings

Calories: 323
Exchanges: *2   Meat*
                 2   Bread
                 ½   Milk

Cholesterol: *27   Mg*
SF: *1   Gm*
Fat: *5   Gm*
Sodium: *656 Mg*
Dietary Fiber: *3   Gm*

CHICKEN AND DRESSING - TRADITIONAL RECIPE

CORNBREAD:

2	cups cornmeal
¾	cup all purpose flour
2⅕	teaspoons baking powder
¾	teaspoon baking soda
1	tablespoon sugar
1	cup diced celery
½	cup chopped onion
½	teaspoon salt
1	teaspoon black pepper
2¼	cups buttermilk
3	eggs
1	ounce chicken base
8	ounces butter
1	pound cooked chicken parts

CORNBREAD:

Preheat oven to 450 degrees F. Combine cornmeal, flour, baking powder, soda and sugar in bowl. Combine buttermilk and egg. Add to dry ingredients, stirring just until moistened. Prepare 10" cast iron skillet with oil. Pour batter into skillet and bake 25 - 30 minutes or until golden brown. Let cool. Crumble cornbread into fine pieces.

DRESSING:

In a buttered skillet, cook celery and onion over high heat. Transfer to a large mixing bowl. Add crumbled cornbread. Stir in chicken base, broth, eggs, butter, salt, pepper and cooked chicken. Place in a large baking dish. Bake at 400 degrees F for 40 minutes or until lightly browned.

Yield: 8 servings

Calories: 607
Exchanges: 2½ *Meat*
2 *Bread*
5 *Fat*

Cholesterol: 252 *Mg*
SF: 18 *Gm*
Fat: 35 *Gm*
Sodium: 1,272 *Mg*
Dietary Fiber: 3 *Gm*

CORN CASSEROLE - LIGHT RECIPE

1 cup egg substitute
½ cup liquid Butter Buds
¾ cup cornmeal
1 teaspoon baking powder
½ teaspoon garlic powder
1 chopped jalapeno pepper
1 cup grated light cheddar cheese
2 cans low sodium creamed style corn
   vegetable cooking spray

Combine egg substitute, butter substitute, cornmeal, baking powder, garlic, jalapenos, creamed corn and grated cheese. Place in casserole dish prepared with non-stick vegetable spray. Bake at 350 degrees F for 45 minutes.

Yield: 8 servings

Calories: 232
Exchanges: *1*   *Meat*
                 2   *Bread*
                 <1 *Fat*

Cholesterol: *15* *Mg*
SF: *2*   *Gm*
Fat: *5*   *Gm*
Sodium: *669* *Mg*
Dietary Fiber: *2*   *Gm*

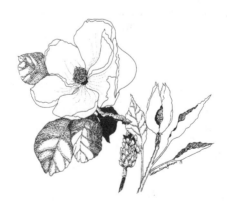

CORN CASSEROLE - TRADITIONAL RECIPE

¾ cup cornmeal
1 teaspoon baking powder
½ teaspoon garlic powder
2 tablespoons chopped jalapeno peppers
3 cups canned sweet corn
4 eggs
4 tablespoons butter
8 ounces cheddar cheese, shredded

Combine eggs, butter, cornmeal, baking powder, garlic. Put in casserole prepared with non-stick vegetable spray. Bake at 350 degrees F for 45 minutes.

Yield: 8 servings

Calories: 345
Exchanges: 1 *Meat*
2 *Bread*
3 *Fats*

Cholesterol: 152 *Mg*
SF: 11 *Gm*
Fat: 19 *Gm*
Sodium: 333 *Mg*
Dietary Fiber: 2 *Gm*

LIGHT AND CRISPY ENCHILADA CASSEROLE

1	6 ounce can tomato paste
½	cup water
1	cup fat free cheddar cheese grated
1	16 ounce can of kidney beans
3	tablespoons chili powder
1	teaspoon cumin
1	teaspoon garlic powder
1	cup chopped onion
6	corn tortillas
1	cup fat free sour cream
1	14 ounce jar enchilada sauce
1	pound Healthy Choice ground beef
	vegetable cooking spray

Brown meat, onions and seasonings. Drain and wash kidney beans. Bake tortillas in 350 degree F oven until crispy, about 15 minutes. Combine meat, kidney beans with ½ cup cheese and enchilada sauce tomato paste, water and three crumbled tortillas. Pour into oblong cooking baking dish that has been sprayed with cooking spray. Bake uncovered at 375 degrees F for 30 minutes. Spread sour cream over top, sprinkle with ½ cup cheese. Make a circle of the 3 crushed tortillas remaining. Bake an additional 5 minutes.

Yield: 6 servings

Calories: 300
Exchanges: 3 *Meat*
             2 *Bread*
             2 *Veg*

Cholesterol: 50 *Mg*
SF: 1 *Gm*
Fat: 4 *Gm*
Sodium: 862 *Mg*
Dietary Fiber: 7 *Gm*

ENCHILADA CASSEROLE - TRADITIONAL RECIPE

6	ounces tomato paste
½	cups water
1	can (16 ounces) kidney beans
1	can (16 ounces) stewed tomatoes
3	tablespoons chili powder
1	teaspoon cumin
1	teaspoon garlic powder
1	cup chopped onion
8	ounces crushed corn chips
1	jar (14 ounces) enchilada sauce
8	ounces cheddar cheese
8	ounces sour cream
1	pound ground beef

Combine 1½ cups grated cheese, enchilada sauce, meat that has been browned with onions and seasonings, tomato paste, water, onion and ½ of the crumbled corn chips. Pour into an oblong baking dish prepared with vegetable spray. Bake uncovered at 375 degrees F for 30 minutes. Spread sour cream over the top. Sprinkle with ½ cup cheese. Use remaining crushed corn chips to circle on the top. Bake 5 minutes more.

Yield: 8 servings

Calories: 603
Exchanges: 2 *Meat*
              2 *Bread*
              4 *Fat*

Cholesterol: 92 *Mg*
SF: 11 *Gm*
Fat: 34 *Gm*
Sodium: 906 *Mg*
Dietary Fiber: 9 *Gm*

POT ROAST - LIGHT RECIPE

2	pounds beef eye of round
⅛	teaspoon salt
⅛	teaspoon black pepper
8 - 10	new potatoes
3	ribs of celery, cut in large pieces
3	cups peeled and cubed carrots
1	cup brewed coffee
2	tablespoons cornstarch

Salt and pepper roast and place in a Dutch oven. Pour 1 cup of liquid coffee over roast. Place potatoes, carrots, and celery on sides of roast. Cover and cook for 2 hours or until meat is tender/done. Remove roast and vegetables. Place broth in freezer for several minutes until fat rises to top. Skim off fat. Thicken broth with cornstarch. Add meat back to gravy and heat thoroughly.

Yield: 8 (4 ounces roast with 1 cup vegetables) servings

Calories: 280

Exchanges:	*4*	*Meat*
	1	*Bread*
	2½	*Veg*

Cholesterol:	*79*	*Mg*
SF:	*2*	*Gm*
Fat:	*6*	*Gm*
Sodium:	*155*	*Mg*
Dietary Fiber:	*2*	*Gm*

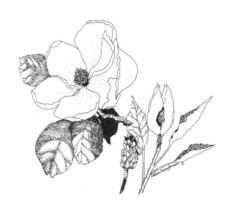

POT ROAST - TRADITIONAL RECIPE

2   pounds chuck roast
2   tablespoons vegetable oil
1   can cream of mushroom soup
1   envelope onion soup mix
1¼ cups water
6 - 8   medium potatoes
3   cups peeled and sliced carrots
2   tablespoons all purpose flour

Brown roast in oil in Dutch oven. Add mushrooms soup, soup mix and 1 cup water to roast. Simmer covered for 2 hours. Add potatoes and carrots and cook covered for 45 minutes. Remove roast and vegetables to serving platter. Mix flour and ¼ cup cold water to form a smooth paste. Add to pan liquids. Stir continuously until thickened over high heat. Serve gravy with roast and vegetables.

Yield: 8 (4 ounces roast with 1 cup vegetables) servings

Calories: 389
Exchanges: *3   Meat*
                1   Bread
                2   Veg
                1   Fat

Cholesterol: *69 Mg*
SF: *8   Gm*
Fat: *23 Gm*
Sodium: *405 Mg*
Dietary Fiber: *3   Gm*

SEAFOOD CASSEROLE - LIGHT RECIPE

1   can Healthy Request cream of mushroom soup
¼   cup skim milk
¼   cup egg substitute
4   tablespoons fat free Parmesan cheese
½   pound fresh crab meat
6   ounces raw shrimp, peeled
½   cup chopped mushrooms
½   cup bread crumbs
1   teaspoon dry butter substitute

Combine soup, milk, egg substitute and 2 tablespoons fat free Parmesan cheese. Sauté shrimp, crab and mushrooms in a skillet sprayed with cooking spray until shrimp are pink. Combine all ingredients and place in a casserole dish prepared with vegetable cooking spray. Combine bread crumbs, butter substitute and remaining Parmesan cheese. Bake at 375 degrees F for 30 minutes or until bread crumbs are browned and casserole is bubbly.

Yield: 6 servings

Calories: 105
Exchanges: *2*   *Meat*
               ½   *Bread*

Cholesterol: *70*   *Mg*
SF: *<1*   *Gm*
Fat: *1*   *Gm*
Sodium: *327* *Mg*
Dietary Fiber: *<1* *Gm*

SEAFOOD CASSEROLE - TRADITIONAL RECIPE

- ¼ **cup milk**
- ½ **pound crab meat**
- 6 **ounces shrimp**
- ½ **cup chopped mushrooms**
- 1 **can cream of mushroom soup**
- 1 **egg**
- 4 **tablespoons grated Parmesan cheese**
- 4 **tablespoons butter**
- ½ **cup bread crumbs**

Combine cream soup, milk, egg and 2 tablespoons Parmesan cheese. Sauté shrimp, crab and mushrooms in butter shrimp are pink. Combine all ingredients and place in a casserole dish prepared with butter. Combine bread crumbs, butter and remaining Parmesan cheese. Bake at 375 degrees F for 30 minutes or until bread crumbs are browned and casserole is bubbly.

Yield: 6 servings

Calories: 233
Exchanges: 2   *Meat*
                3   *Fat*

Cholesterol: *158 Mg*
SF: 7   *Gm*
Fat: 15   *Gm*
Sodium: *758 Mg*
Dietary Fiber: 0   *Gm*

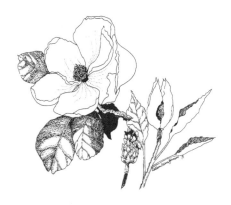

SEAFOOD GUMBO - LIGHT RECIPE

½ cup fat free roux
4   ribs of celery, diced
2   cups onion, chopped
½ cup bell pepper
½ pound okra
2   quarts fat free chicken broth
1   quart water
¼ cup Worcestershire sauce
1   teaspoon Tabasco sauce
16 ounce can stewed tomatoes
1   teaspoon salt
4   ounces Healthy Choice ham
1   bay leaf
¼ thyme
½ rosemary
¼ red pepper
32 ounces shrimp, peeled and deveined
8   ounces cooked, skinned chicken breast, diced
16 ounces crab meat
    vegetable cooking spray

Spray large cooking pot with cooking spray. Heat and add celery, onion, green peppers and garlic. Cook 25 minutes over low heat. Sprinkle with fat free roux (refer to index for recipe.) Add okra. Cook 2 to 3 minutes. Add broth, water, Worcestershire sauce, hot sauce, stewed tomatoes, salt, ham, thyme, rosemary, bay leaf and cayenne pepper. Simmer 2½ hours. Stir occasionally. Add shrimp, chicken and crab during the last 10 minutes of simmering period. Remove bay leaf. Serve over rice and sprinkle with gumbo file if desired.

Yield: 16 (1 cup) servings

Calories: 164
Exchanges: 3   *Meat*
                  1   *Veg*

Cholesterol: 116 *Mg*
SF: <1 *Gm*
Fat: 3   *Gm*
Sodium: 798 *Mg*
Dietary Fiber: 1   *Gm*

SEAFOOD GUMBO - TRADITIONAL RECIPE

1   cup butter
2   cups all purpose flour
6   quarts water
1   can (10 ounces) Rotel tomatoes with chilies
1   cup diced celery
3   cups chopped onion
1   cup chopped bell pepper
4   pounds shrimp
1   pound fresh crab meat
6   raw oysters
¼   teaspoon red pepper

Make a dark brown roux with butter and flour. Add water. Bring to a boil and cook until roux is dissolved. Reduce heat. Add tomatoes with chilies, celery, onions, bell pepper and garlic. Simmer on low 1 - 3 hours. Add shrimp and simmer 10 minutes. Add crab meat, oysters, salt, pepper and red pepper. Simmer 10 -15 minutes. Serve 1 cup of gumbo over ⅓ cup rice.

Yield: 12 servings

Calories: 556
Exchanges: 5   *Meat*
              1½ *Bread*
               4   *Fat*

Cholesterol: *381 Mg*
SF: *13 Gm*
Fat: *25 Gm*
Sodium: *810 Mg*
Dietary Fiber: 2   *Gm*

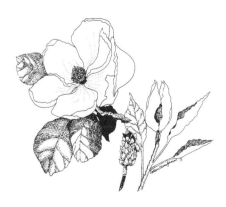

NUTRITIONAL INFORMATION

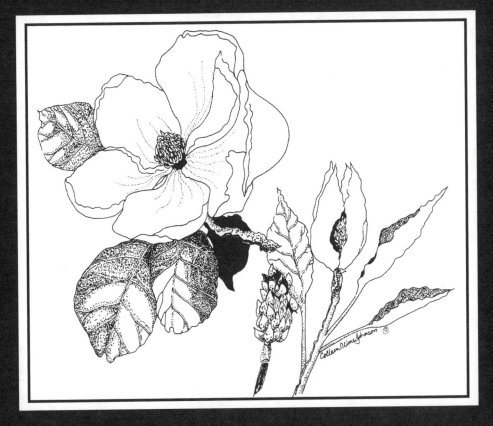

GOAL WEIGHT

In determining goal weight, there are many factors to be considered. Be realistic, remember genetics play a large part in one's appearance. Are your parents overweight? Your medical history is very important. Are you physically active? Try to set a goal weight you have maintained in the past and at which you were comfortable.

A nutritionist may help you determine goal weight, appropriate calorie level and monitor your weight, and advise you on how to make the proper adjustments in calories and fat.

Formula to determine goal weight:

Based on Height:

For 5 feet, allow 100 pounds	100
For every inch over 5 feet, add 5 pounds	_____
For every inch under 5 feet, subtract 5 pounds	_____
Goal Weight	_____

Adjust weight for Body Frame:

For large frame, add 5-10 pounds	_____
For small frame, subtract 5-10 pounds	_____
Adjusted Goal weight	_____

*Most people are medium frame and need no adjustment.

DETERMINE YOUR CALORIE LEVEL

Formula to Determine Calories/Day
Goal Weight X 10 equals Calories/Day
(Sedentary Person)

If you are lightly active, add:	10% more calories each day
moderately active, add:	20% more calories each day
extremely active, add:	30% more calories each day

Most people are generally sedentary. Exercise is a necessary component to any weight loss or maintenance program. We recommend walking as a good low impact exercise. Warming up and cooling down are important for everyone. Check with your physician before starting any exercise program.

Quick Referenced for Calorie Selection
(General Recommendations)

	MEN	**WOMEN**
Height	5'4" - 5'10"	5'0" - 5'5"
Present Wt.	160 - 200	120 - 150
Calories	1500 - 1700	1000 - 1200
Height	5'11" - 6'4"	5'6" - 6'0"
Present Wt.	200 -300	160 - 200
Calories	1700 - 2000	1200 - 1500

Formula to Determine Fat Grams

The American Heart Association recommends that 30% of an average individual's calories be derived from fat. However, if you are presently on a high fat diet, you may wish to begin with 30%, lowering the fat content as you lose weight. If any genetic conditions predispose you to heart disease, diabetes, or cancer, you may wish to consult your physician and follow a lower fat diet.

Refer to the following chart:

Grams of fat per day based on calories/percentage of fat

Calories	10%	20%	30%
1200	13	27	40
1500	17	33	50
2000	22	44	66
2500	28	56	83
3000	33	67	100

My allowed fat grams are: _____

Getting Started

Fat Gram Sheets have been prepared to aid in your calculations. Document all foods eaten during the day. Do not exceed your fat gram allowance. For your convenience all foods in "bold" print are the best selections to use.

FAT GRAM SHEET
(APPROXIMATE FAT GRAMS)

EXTRA LEAN MEATS, POULTRY & FISH - 1 GM FAT
or less (per ounce)

FISH: Catfish, Water packed tuna, Flounder, Cod, Haddock, Pollack, Perch, Red Snapper, Swordfish, Sturgeon, Sole, Pink Salmon, Flounder, Bass

***SHELL FISH: Lobster, Crawfish, Scallops, Oysters, Shrimp, Crab**

****POULTRY: Chicken Breast, Turkey Breast, Lean deli sliced Turkey and Chicken**

RED MEAT: Healthy Choice Hamburger, ***Healthy Choice Wieners - 93 to 98 per cent fat free, Lean sliced deli ham

VENISON (not mixed with sausage)

* Moderately high in cholesterol, limit one time per week, or as specified by nutritionist.
** All poultry should be skinned before cooking
***Processed meats can be high in sodium and preservatives

LEAN MEATS - 3 GMS. FAT (per ounce)

FISH: Salmon, Atlantic & Chinook, Rainbow Trout, Mackerel

POULTRY: Dark Meat Chicken and Turkey, Commercially Ground Turkey

RED MEAT: Flank Steak, Tenderloin, Round, all cuts Rump, Tripe, Filet, Diet Lean Hamburger

PORK: Lean Ham, Center Cut Chop, Center Shank, Loin

SAUSAGE: Turkey Sausage, Low-Fat or Pork Loin Sausage

MEDIUM FAT MEATS - 5 GMS FAT (per ounce)

BEEF: Ground Round, Corned Beef, Sirloin

PORK: Canadian Bacon, Boiled Ham

VENISON: Mixed with Pork Sausage

FAT MEATS- 8 GMS FAT (per ounce)

POULTRY: Duck, Goose

BEEF: Brisket, Regular Ground Beef, Commercial Hamburger Patties, Chuck Roast, Club Steak

LAMB: Breast

PEANUT BUTTER: 2 Tablespoons: 14 - 16 gms

PORK: Spareribs, Ground Pork, Country Style Ham

COLD CUTS, Luncheon Meats

WIENERS, including many varieties of chicken and turkey wieners

MILK AND DAIRY PRODUCTS: (TRACE OF FAT)

MILK: Skimmed: 1 Cup
Powdered, (⅓ Cup Non-Fat Dry before adding liquid in 8 oz. Glass)

BUTTERMILK from skim milk - 1 cup

CHEESE: Fat Free Cottage, ¼ Cup Fat Free, per ounce American, Cheddar, Swiss, Mozzarella, Parmesan, Ricotta

PLAIN YOGURT: (Unflavored from skim milk)

SKIM/CANNED EVAPORATED

FAT FREE SOUR CREAM

FAT FREE YOGURT

MILK AND DAIRY PRODUCTS: 3 GMS FAT

1% MILK: 1 Cup

PARMESAN CHEESE: 1 Tablespoon

MILK AND DAIRY PRODUCTS: 5 GMS FAT

2% MILK: 1 Cup
YOGURT (FROM 2% MILK): 1 Cup
EGG: 1

CHEESE PER OUNCE: Mozzarella, Ricotta, Farmer's, Neufchatel, Parmesan

MILK AND DAIRY PRODUCTS: 8 GMS FAT

WHOLE MILK: 1 Cup
BUTTERMILK (FROM WHOLE MILK): 1 Cup
CANNED EVAPORATED MILK: ½ Cup

CHEESE PER OUNCE: Cheddar
YOGURT (FROM WHOLE MILK): 1 Cup

STARCHES OR BREADS: 0 - 1 GM FAT

White, Wheat Bread - 1 Slice
English Muffin - 1
Plain Roll - 1
Hamburger Bun - ½
Bagels - ½
*Unsweetened cereal (Bran Flakes, Cornflakes) - ¾ Cup
Cooked cereal - ½ cup
Air Popped Popcorn - 3 Cups
Fat Free Pretzels - 1 ounce
Low Fat Biscuits - 1
Frozen Fat Free Waffle

Pasta - ½ Cup
Cornmeal - 2 Tablespoons
Flour - 2½ Tablespoons
Graham Crackers - 2
Crackers, Fat Free - 8
Peas & Beans - ½ Cup
Corn - ⅓ Cup
Potato - 1 Small
Rice - ½ Cup
Fat Free Flour Tortilla
Low Fat Tortilla Chips 12 - 14

STARCHES OR BREADS: 5 GMS FAT

Biscuit: 2"
Cornbread: 2"x 2"
Waffle: 1

Potato Chips: 15 (10 to 14 gms)
Corn Muffin: 2¼"
Pancake: 1

FATS - 0 GMS FAT

Fat Free Mayonnaise - 1 Tablespoon   Fat Free Salad Dressings - 1 Tablespoon

FATS - 3 GMS FAT

Lite Mayonnaise - 1 Tablespoon   Lite Salad Dressing - 1 Tablespoon

FATS - 5 GMS FAT

Butter - Soft, Tub, Stick - 1½ Teaspoons
Margarine - Soft, Tub, Stick - 1½ Teaspoons
Avocado - ⅛
Oils (Corn, Cottonseed, Safflower, Canola, Sunflower) - 1½ Teaspoons
Olive Oil - 1½ Teaspoons
Peanut Oil - 1½ Teaspoons

Almonds - 10 Whole
Pecans - 2 Large Whole
Walnuts - 6 small
Other nuts - 6 small
Salad Dressing - 1 Teaspoon
Mayonnaise - 2 Teaspoons
Salad Dressings - 1 Tablespoon
Sour Cream - 2 Tablespoons

VEGETABLES - 0 GMS FAT (½ cup of each)

Asparagus
Bean Sprouts
Broccoli
Brussels Sprouts
Cabbage
Carrots
Cauliflower
Celery

Eggplant
Green Pepper
Greens
Vegetable Juice
Turnips
Zucchini
Yellow Squash
Rutabaga
Green Beans

Chinese Cabbage
Lettuce
Parsley
Radishes
Watercress
Escarole
Endive
Cucumbers
Tomatoes

FRUITS- O GMS FAT

Apple - 1 Small
Apple Juice - ⅓ Cup
Banana - ½ Cup
Berries - ½ Cup
Strawberries - ¾ Cup
Cantaloupe - ¼ Small
Grapes - 12
Grape Juice - ¼ Cup
Kiwi - 1
Nectarine - 1
Orange - 1 Small

Orange Juice - ½ Cup
Peach - 1 Medium
Pear - 1 Small
Pineapple - ½ Cup
Figs - 2
Prune Juice - ¼ Cup
Prunes - 2 Medium
Tangerine - 1 Medium
Watermelon - 1 Cup
Plums - 2

CONDIMENTS: 0 GMS FAT

Salsa	Herbs	Non-stick Vegetable
Mustard	Spices	Sprays
Pepper	Lemon	Sugar Substitutes
Molly McButter	Lemon Juice	Reduced Sodium Soy
Butter Buds	Vinegar	Sauce

BEVERAGES

Coffee	Quest Beverages	Sugar free Apple Cider
Tea	Sugar free/Fat free Hot	Mix
	Chocolate	

EXAMPLE: <40 GMS FAT*

Breakfast:
  1 Fruit
  ½ Cup Cereal
  1 Cup 2% Milk (5 gms.)
  Coffee or Tea

Lunch:
  2 ounces Meat (lean) - (6 gms.)
  2 Starches
  1 Cup Vegetable/1 Salad
  1 Fruit
  1 Teaspoon Mayonnaise (5 gms.)

Dinner:
  4 ounces Meat (lean) - (12 gms)
  2 Starches
  1 Cup Vegetable/Salad
  Salad
  1 Fruit
  1 Teaspoon Margarine - (5 gms)
  1 Cup 2% milk - (5 gms)

Snack:
  1 ounce Fat Free Cheese
  6-8 Fat Free Crackers

*35 gms. fat, allowing for medium fat
meat one or two times per week.

EXAMPLE: <20 GMS FAT*

Breakfast:
  1 Fruit
  ½ Cup Cereal
  1 Cup Skimmed milk
  Coffee or Tea

Lunch:
  2 ounces Meat (extra - lean) -
    (2 gms.)
  1 Starch
  1 Cup Vegetable/1 Salad
  1 Fruit

Dinner:
  4 oz Meat (lean) - (12 gms)
  1 Starch
  1 Cup Vegetable/Salad
  Salad
  1 Fruit
  1 Cup Skimmed milk

Snack:
  Air Popped Popcorn
  Fruit

*25 gms fat, allowing for medium fat
meat one or two times per week.

REMEMBER!!

Read labels: Fat varies depending on brand. (See label information). Try to use extra lean meats and non fat dairy sources as much as possible when selecting protein choices.

Eating Out: Allow 5 grams additional fat per serving of vegetables, baked, broiled, grilled, lean meat, poultry and starch when eating out. Eating out daily is difficult for anyone on a low fat program. Many times hidden fats make a difference in having successful results.

Fluid: Water is an important tool during weight loss. Two (2) quarts a day is recommended for most people.

Prepared Foods: Be careful. Many prepared foods are high fat. Read labels and choose frozen dinners and entrees with no more than 30% fat. Adding vegetables, fruits and non fat dairy products to these meals satisfy without adding fat.

3 DAY MENU PLAN
20 Grams fat per day

Breakfast

2 Ballard Light Biscuits
1 Tablespoon Fat Free
Margarine
1 Tablespoon Low Sugar
Jam
1 Cup Skim Milk
Coffee / Hot Tea

Lunch

* 1½ Cups Seafood
Gumbo
8 Fat Free Crackers
Salad
Fat Free Dressing
1 Fresh Fruit
Iced Tea / Water

Dinner

* Light Crispy Enchilada
Casserole
Vegetable Salad
Fat Free Dressing
1 ounce Baked Tortilla
Chips
1 Fresh Fruit
Iced Tea / Water

Snack

8 ounces Non-fat Yogurt

Breakfast

1 Eggbeater Cooked
with Pam
2 Slices Toast /
1 Tablespoon Fat Free
Margarine
½ Cup Orange Juice
Coffee / Hot Tea

Lunch

* 1 Cup Hot Chicken
Salad
1 Cup Raw Vegetables
1 Fresh Fruit
Iced Tea / Water

Dinner

* 1 Cup Meat Sauce /
1 Cup Spaghetti
Salad / Fat Free Dressing
2 - 1 Inch Slices French
Bread
Butter Flavored Cooking
Spray / Garlic
1 Fresh Fruit
Iced Tea / Water

Snack

1 Fresh Fruit

Breakfast

2 Slices Bread
1 Slice Fat Free Cheese
Cooking Spray (to make
grilled cheese)
½ Cup Orange Juice
Coffee / Hot Tea /
Sugar-Free Hot Cocoa

Lunch

3 ounces Healthy Choice
Hamburger / Bun
Fat Free Mayonnaise /
Mustard
Lettuce / Tomato
1 ounce Pretzels
1 Fresh Fruit
Iced Tea / Water

Dinner

* Oven Fried Fish
* Oven Fries
* Jack's Polka Dot Slaw
2 Tablespoons Catsup
1 Fresh Fruit
Iced Tea / Water

Snack

1 Cup Raw Vegetables

3 DAY MENU PLAN
40 Grams fat per day

Breakfast

Blueberry Bagel
1 Cup 2% Milk
2 Tablespoons Fat Free
Cream Cheese
Coffee / Hot Tea

Lunch

2 Slices Bread
2 ounces Lean Ham
1 Slice Fat Free Cheese
1 Tablespoon Fat Free
Mayonnaise
11 Mr. Phipp's Tator
Chips
1 Fresh Fruit
Iced Tea / Water

Dinner

4 ounces Lean Pork Loin
Chop
* ½ Cup Corn Casserole
1 Cup Steamed Green
Beans
1 Roll
1 Fresh Fruit
1 Cup 2% Milk

Snack

3 Cups Air Popped Popcorn

Breakfast

2 Fat Free Waffles
2 Tablespoons Light
Syrup /
1 Tablespoon Fat Free
Margarine
1 Cup 2% Milk
Coffee / Hot Tea

Lunch

* 1½ Cups Homestyle
Chili
8 Fat Free Saltines
Salad
2 Tablespoons Fat Free
Dressing
1 Fresh Fruit
Iced Tea / Water

Dinner

* Seafood Casserole
Salad / 2 Tablespoons
Fat Free Dressing
2 Slices French Bread
Butter Flavored Pam /
Garlic Powder
* 1 Slice Fat Free
Carrot Cake
Iced Tea / Water

Snack

1 Cup 2% Milk / 1 Fresh Fruit

Breakfast

¾ Cup Fat Free Granola
Cereal
1 Fresh Fruit
1 Cup 2% Milk
Coffee / Hot Tea

Lunch

* 1½ Cups Grilled
Chicken Pasta Salad
8 Fat Free Saltines
1 Cup Raw Vegetables
1 Fresh Fruit
Iced Tea / Water

Dinner

* 4 ounces Oven Fried
Chicken
* ½ Cup Creamed
Potatoes
1 Cup Steamed Broccoli
1 Roll
Fat Free Yogurt with
¾ Cup Strawberries
Iced Tea / Water

Snack

1 Slice Fat Free Cheese / 6 Fat Free Saltines

TROUBLE SHOOTER GUIDE

If you are not seeing good results for weight loss, first recommit to staying with the program.

Weigh all meats, try to stay with extra lean meats having 1 gram of fat per ounce

Measure all foods

Do not use added margarines or oil. (Use only butter substitutes)

Limit red meats one time a week

Drink plenty of water (2 quarts per day)

Exercise - walk 20-30 minutes daily minimum (Always check with a physician before starting any exercise program)

Use low fat cooking methods

Avoid sugar (Sugar can make you hungry and cause fluid retention)

Limit eating out

Discontinue snacking

Increase exercise level

Get back to basic foods (Lean meat, starch, vegetable, salad, fresh fruit)

Limit sodium - possibly fluid retention

Most women may see fluid retention at some time during their cycle

Medications can affect weight loss, blood lipids and fluid retention. (Check with your physician)

NATIONAL CENTER FOR NUTRITION AND DIETETICS

Nutrition
FACT·SHEET

INTRODUCING THE NEW FOOD LABEL IN BITE-SIZE PIECES

Have you seen the new food labels?

Feast your eyes on the new food labels designed to give you the information you need to make healthful food choices wherever you buy food. With the new food labels, you can use the information to make more informed food choices. Since the new food labels show you how to balance the nutrients you need each day, choosing a variety of great tasting food has never been easier.

What should you look at first?

The new food labels offer a full course of information, so don't try to digest it all at once. For starters, sink your teeth into four bite-size pieces listed under the new heading "Nutrition Facts."

■ **Set priorities**
The "Nutrition Facts" panel makes it easy to apply key nutrition and health issues to food choices. Now you'll be able to find information on fat, cholesterol, sodium, fiber, and other food components that may help reduce the risk of heart disease,

Nutrition Facts

Serving Size 1 cup (227 g)
Servings Per Container 1

Amount Per Serving

Calories 100   Calories from Fat 0

	% Daily Value*
Total Fat 0 g	0%
Saturated Fat 0 g	0%
Cholesterol <5 mg	2%
Sodium 140 mg	6%
Total Carbohydrate 17 g	6%
Dietary Fiber 0 g	0%
Sugars 13 g	
Protein 9 g	

Vitamin A 0%	•	Vitamin C 0%
Calcium 30%	•	Iron 4%

*Percent Daily Values are based on a 2,000 calorie diet. Your daily values may be higher or lower depending on your calorie needs.

some types of cancer and other chronic diseases. The information you see here will appear on most food labels under the heading "Nutrition Facts."

■ **Size up the food**
Now it's easier to use this information because serving sizes are listed in household measures. Also, the serving size listed on the product represents the amount that most people typically eat. When interpreting the nutrition information, be sure to personalize the product serving size to the amount you actually eat.

■ **Scan calories and calories from fat**
Calories and calories from fat are two important aspects of every food. You can use this information to help you balance your food choices.

■ **Check the vitamins and minerals**
Vitamins A and C, and the minerals calcium and iron may be listed on the new label. Your goal is a daily total of 100% of each vitamin and mineral for all the foods you eat in a day.

Does the "Total Fat" value incorporate all types of fat including saturated fat?

The total fat value includes all types of fat—saturated fat, as well as, polyunsaturated and monounsaturated. While many factors affect heart disease, diets low in saturated fat and cholesterol may decrease the risk of this disease. The new food label enables you to balance higher fat food choices with lower fat choices, making it easy to enjoy a variety of great tasting foods.

If a food product contains no added sugar, why is sugar listed under carbohydrates?

Sugars are found naturally in foods like fruits, vegetables, milk, cereals, grains and legumes. Sugar may also be added during processing in the form of sucrose, high fructose corn syrup or honey. The "sugars" category on the new food label includes both the naturally occurring and added sugar content of the food.

In addition, you may have noticed that the components under total carbohydrate don't always equal the number listed for total carbohydrate. That's because total carbohydrate includes sugar, starches and some fiber which, depending on the food product, may or may not be listed on the label.

Serving up the rest of the food label

Once you have whet your appetite with the first part of the food label, you are ready for the next course. Here is an overview of additional food label information and how it may assist you in your daily meal planning.

Let the % Daily Value be your guide

The % Daily Value gives you a general idea of a food's nutrient contribution to a 2,000 calorie reference diet. Your specific dietary needs may differ depending on your calorie intake.

Look for nutrient content claims on the front of the package

Food companies may use descriptive terms like "low fat" or "sugar free" to help guide your food choices. Descriptive terms must meet strictly defined government standards. For example, if a food claims to be low calorie, you can be assured that the product has 40 calories or less per serving.

It's what's inside that counts

The ingredient list tells you exactly what's in a food. Ingredients are listed by weight from most to least - those in largest amounts are listed first, near the beginning of the list. For example, bread that lists "wheat flour" first on the ingredient list means that wheat flour is the main ingredient in the food.

All foods can be incorporated into a healthy lifestyle. The new food label offers a smorgasbord of information to help you stay healthy while choosing a variety of great tasting foods.

For more information
■ **The American Dietetic Association/National Center For Nutrition and Dietetics.** For answers to your food and nutrition questions and to get a referral to a registered dietitian in your area call the Consumer Nutrition Hot Line 800/366-1655, 9 am-4 pm (Central Time), Monday-Friday.

■ E-Z Food Labels Survival Guide. The NutraSweet Company, 1994. Write to: **The NutraSweet Company, 1751 Lake Cook Road, Box 830, Deerfield, IL 60015.**

©ADAF 1994
This fact sheet is supported by an educational grant from The NutraSweet Company. The ADA does not endorse the services or products of any company.

NATIONAL CENTER FOR NUTRITION AND DIETETICS
of The American Dietetic Association
216 West Jackson Boulevard • Chicago, Illinois 60606-6995
312/899-0040, Ext. 4653 • FAX 312/899-1739

FOOD PRODUCTS

The following products are generally available at most grocery stores.

MEATS

Healthy Choice ground beef - 1 gram of fat per ounce

Bryan light ground sausage - a blend of pork loin or turkey

Healthy Choice and Hormel light wieners - about 1 gram of fat each

Healthy Choice low fat sausages

Healthy Choice, Louis Rich, Hillshire's Farms, and Bryan - lean sliced turkey, chicken breasts and ham

Peter Eckrich deli light roast beef, 1 gram of fat per ounce

Tyson - frozen grilled chicken breast portions, great for a quick lunch on a hamburger bun

CHEESES

Weight Watchers Parmesan cheese - fat free

Healthy Choice and Alpine Lace fat free cheeses - American, cheddar, Swiss, Mozzarella, string cheese, soft cheeses

Healthy Choice fat free cream cheese - also available in a strawberry flavor. Great on a bagel

Philadelphia fat free cream cheese

Kraft and Borden fat free singles - American, Swiss and cheddar

Kraft Light Naturals - reduced fat, use sparingly, melts better than fat free cheeses

Sargento low fat Ricotta

Frigo fat free Ricotta

Light and Lively, Borden and some generic brands - fat free cottage cheese (may be substituted for Ricotta)

COOKING PRODUCTS

Healthy Choice, Hunts, Campbell's Healthy Request and other - fat free spaghetti sauces

Campbell's Healthy Request and Healthy Choice soups

Avis and Ward fat free soup bases - Information available upon request.

Land O Lakes - fat free sour cream

Egg Beaters, Better N Eggs - fat free, cholesterol free egg substitute (2 egg whites can be substituted for one whole egg)

Pet skimmed evaporated milk

Pioneer fat free biscuit mix - great to make low fat pancakes, waffles and biscuits

Healthline hamburger and hot dog buns

MARGARINE, CONDIMENTS AND DRESSINGS

Promise Ultra fat free margarine - does not melt well, good to use as a spread

Smart Beat light margarine - 2 grams fat per tablespoon

Weight Watchers extra light low fat margarine - 4 grams per tablespoon

Butter Buds - butter substitute, can be used in dry form or mixed with water, 0 fat

Fat Free mayonnaise - most national brands

Fat Free salad dressing - most national brands

Vegetable cooking sprays - national brands and generic

Salsa - most brands are fat free

SNACKS

Be careful when choosing snacks not to overload your diet with a lot of high sugar products. Read labels. Low fat snacks should be incorporated into a balanced meal plan. Eating too many low fat and fat free snacks may prevent weight loss and possibly cause weight gain. Calories still must be balanced with exercise.

Yoplait, Dannon, Weight Watchers - non fat yogurts, many fruit varieties and plain available

Pop Weavers light, Act II low fat popcorn - have average of 3 grams of fat per 3 cups

Minute Maid - juice pops

Quaker rice cakes - various flavors, avoid too many high sugar snacks

Nabisco fat free fig newtons

Snackwell low fat and fat free products

Health Valley low fat and fat free products

Fat free crackers - most national brands

Blue Bell, Healthy Choice, Guilt Free (Yarnell) - fat free desserts and ice creams and frozen yogurts

Smucker's - fat free caramel and chocolate ice cream toppings

Pretzels - all major brands have fat free

Nabisco Mr. Phipp's Tator Crisps - 1 ounce equals 2 grams fat (11 chips)

Smart Temptations, Guiltless and Tostitos baked tortilla chips - 1 ounce equals approximately 1 gram fat

Natures Best, Wheat Fields and Lenders - bagels, check for local brands

BEVERAGES

Soft drinks - all national brands

Most flavored waters may be as high in calories as regular soft drinks. Diet beverages are virtually calories free, but avoid an excess of sugar substitutes. Water is still the best source of liquid.

FOODS TO ORDER OUT

APPETIZERS:

Seasonal fresh fruit
Raw vegetables
Clear soup or broth
Fruit Juice
Tomato & vegetable juices

ENTREES:

Baked broiled, grilled lean meats
Fish, chicken (remove skin)
Entrees without butter sauces

VEGETABLES & STARCHES:

Veggies, raw, stir-fried, steamed
Avoid fried vegetables
Baked potatoes without margarine or butter
Rice or pasta without fat

SALADS:

At salad bars use the free veggies as your salad base (lettuce, radishes, cucumbers)
Use plenty of raw veggies
Avoid marinated and mayonnaise based salads
Avoid bacon, croutons, olives, cheese and hard broiled eggs
Ask for salad dressings on the side and use only one tablespoon.
Vinegar and lemon juice may be used rather than dressings.
Mixed pasta and veggies without cream sauces.

FAST FOODS:

Small hamburger/omit mayonnaise
Grilled chicken/bun-omit mayonnaise
Turkey sandwich with mustard
Baked potato with salad-omit margarine.
Chunky chicken salad (not mayonnaise based)/reduced calorie dressings.
Grilled chicken, fajitas or chicken burrito w/o sour cream
Small roast beef sandwich/omit mayonnaise
Roast chicken breast with salad
Boiled shrimp with side salad

ALCOHOL:

Alcohol can change the way the body metabolizes fat, leading to decreased weight loss.

BUFFETS:

All-you-can-eat buffets are often inviting but **beware**, you always feel you have to get your money's worth. Order from the menu!

SUBSTITUTION LIST

FOOD	SUBSTITUTION
Whole milk	Skim, non fat or 1% milk
Bulgarian buttermilk	Buttermilk made from skim or 1% milk
Cream	Skim evaporated milk
Non dairy creamer	Non fat powdered milk
Cream style cottage cheese	Non fat cottage cheese
American cheese	Fat free American, Lite or reduced fat cheese
Mozzarella cheese	Part skim Mozzarella, fat free Mozzarella
Hard cheese	Fat free cheeses or reduced fat cheeses
Egg	¼ cup egg substitute, 2 egg whites
Sour cream	Non fat sour cream or 1 cup non fat yogurt plus 1 tablespoon cornstarch
Mayonnaise	Non fat mayonnaise, non fat yogurt
Butter	Margarines (the softer the better), reduced calorie margarines, butter substitutes
Hamburger/ground chuck	Healthy choice ground beef, ground turkey breast, ground chicken
Bacon	Canadian bacon, lean ham, smoked turkey
Pork chop	Pork cutlet, pork loin
Pork/beef sausage	Ground turkey sausage, lean ground pork sausage
Whole chicken	Chicken breast, skinned
Shortening/lard	Vegetable oils
Oil based marinades	Fat free dressings
Chocolate/cocoa butter	3 tablespoons cocoa plus 1 tablespoon vegetable oil or 3 tablespoons cocoa plus 1 tablespoon margarine
Gravy	Chicken or beef granules (low sodium are available - consult your physician) thickened with cornstarch (see Sauce section of cookbook)
Egg noodles	Plain noodles, spaghetti, macaroni with no added fat

COOKING TIPS

Cut back on margarine and oils in dishes by half or use butter substitutes.

Use low fat white sauces rather than canned soups. (See Sauce Section in cookbook) Try our low fat soup mixes in your favorite recipes. (See the Order Section of the book).

Use defatted broths for gravies. (See Sauce section in the cookbook).

Cook pasta and rice without fat or salt.

Cook vegetables in fat free broths or liquid smoke.

Use herbs and spices along with jalapeno peppers, picante sauce, vinegars, and spicy mustards to replace the flavor of salt and fat.

Use applesauce rather than oil in baked dishes

Omit and add procedures to recipes:

> *Chill stocks to reduce fat
> *Always trim meats
> *Use alternate cooking methods (broil, grill, steam, rather than frying)

Non-stick skillets and non-stick vegetable sprays: Help avoid using excess fat.

Pressure cooker: Saves time and cooks foods quickly.

Wire grilling baskets: Great for grilling fish.

Broiler pan: Helps to cook meats low fat.

Blender: Excellent to puree vegetables to thicken soups.

Gravy Skimmer: Separates excess fat from gravy.

GETTING INTO EXERCISE

Always check with your physician before starting an exercise program.

Start exercising 3 times a week and gradually increase to 5 out of 7 days.

Exercise firms your muscles, burns off extra calories and can help you cope better with daily stress.

REGULAR EXERCISE CAN HELP:

1) bring down blood pressure

2) lower cholesterol by decreased LDL's (bad cholesterol) while building up HDL's (good cholesterol)

3) kick the smoking habit for a fitness habit

4) reduce your weight

If your physician recommends exercise, be sure to warm up at least 5 minutes and cool down to help your body return to normal.

Exercise is an important part of successful weight loss and weight maintenance.

To get the most out of exercise keep up with your heart rate. The Target Heart Rate Zone is important to make sure you are getting the maximum benefits of the exercise without overworking your heart. Your target zone is dependent upon your age. Rates and charts are available through the American Heart Association.

HEART HELPFUL TIPS:

Begin your exercise program slowly. Set goals and work toward them.

Decide on a realistic activity. Switch activities occasionally to keep from getting bored.

An exercise buddy can provide support to stay with it!

Make time for exercise. Make a schedule and stay with it.

Call your local American Heart Association for further information and resources.

THE IMPORTANCE OF WATER
5 REASONS FOR DRINKING WATER

1.   Water naturally suppresses the appetite.

2.   Water acts as a natural diuretic.
     When the body does not get enough water the kidneys will cause the body to retain fluid. By drinking more water the sodium becomes diluted and causes the kidneys to flush fluid from the body.

3.   Water helps prevents constipation.
     Without an adequate amount of water, the colon becomes dry, preventing normal bowel function. Drinking more water can cause normal bowel functions to return.

4.   Water helps to maintain proper muscle tone.
     Water aids muscles in their natural ability to contract and prevents dehydration.

5.   Water plays a major role in healthy skin.
     It can aid sagging skin following weight loss by shrinking cells that are buoyed by water. Water helps pump the skin, leaving it clear, healthy and resilient.

How much water is enough? The average individual should drink at least 2 quarts or 8 cups per day. For each 25 pounds that an individual is overweight, an additional 8 ounces should be added per day.

EQUIVALENTS

3	teaspoons	1	tablespoon
4	tablespoons	¼	cup
5⅓	tablespoons	⅓	cup
8	tablespoons	½	cup
10⅔	tablespoons	⅔	cup
2	tablespoons	¾	cup
2	cups	1	pint
4	cups	1	quart
4	quarts	1	gallon
32	fluid ounces	1	quart
8	fluid ounces	1	cup
1	fluid ounce	2	tablespoons
16	ounces	1	pound
28.35	ounces	1	gram

INDEX BY FOOD GROUPS

APPETIZERS

Artichoke Dip 12
Brandied Meatballs 15
Broccoli Cheese Bars 10
Cheese Ball 11
Cocktail Meatballs 16
Light Crab Dip 13
Meat Pies 17
Picante Dip 14
Pizza Snack 19
Shrimp Cocktail for a Crowd 20
Spinach and Cheese Dip 13
Stuffed Mushrooms 18
Tex Mex Dip 14

BEEF

Beef and Snow Peas 126
Beef Pot Pie 127
Beef Potluck Casserole 128
Brandied Meatballs 15
Cocktail Meatballs 16
Deep Dish Pizza 139
Easy Lasagne 133
Enchilada Casserole - Traditional Recipe 255
Gravy for Chicken or Beef 31
Grilled Hamburger with Cheese 130
Hamburger Pie 131
Hamburger Stroganoff 132
Homestyle Chili 129
Light and Crispy Enchilada Casserole 254
Louisiana Chicken Jambalaya 106
Mama B's Spaghetti 143
Meat Pies 17
Meatballs and Spaghetti 135
Meatloaf 136
Mexican Lasagna 134
Ole South Coating Mix 30
Pigs in a Blanket 137
Pizza Casserole 138
Pizza Roll 140
Pot Roast - Light Recipe 256
Pot Roast - Traditional Recipe 257
South of the Border Pizza 141
Sportsman's Sauce 33
Steak and Gravy 144

BEEF (Continued)

Steak on a Stick 145
Sunday Roast 142
Sweet and Sour Marinade 31
Tamale Pie 146

BEVERAGES

Café Viennese 21
Deep South Wassail 24
Muscadine Wine 24
Old-Fashioned Strawberry Soda 22
Orange Cappuccino 21
Quick Fruit Punch 23
Swiss Mocha Coffee 22
White Grape Punch 23

BREADS

Apple Muffins 209
Aunt Era's Dumplings 203
Banana Nut Bread 214
Basic Muffin Mix 209
Beer Bread 197
Blueberry Muffins 210
Braided French Bread 200
Bran Muffins 212
Breakfast Biscuits 196
Breakfast Bread 198
Cinnamon Rolls 215
Cornbread 207
Cranberry Christmas Bread 199
Delicious Yeast Rolls 218
Easy Dinner Rolls 217
Easy Muffins 210
Garlic Bread Sticks 201
Jam Muffins 211
Maple Crumb Coffee Cake 216
Oat Muffins 213
Pecan Muffins 211
Soft Pretzels 202
Sour Cream Biscuits 196
Sourdough Biscuits 205
Sourdough Buttermilk Pancakes 206
Sourdough Starter 204
Spinach Cornbread 208

CAKE

7 Minute Icing 227
Apple Spice Cake 221
Blueberry Batter Cake 222

CAKE (Continued)

Carrot Cake - Light Recipe 242
Carrot Cake - Traditional Recipe 243
Chiffon Cake with Kahlua Frosting 224
Chocolate Snack Cake 223
Fat Free Cheese Cake 244
Fresh Apple Cake 220
New York Cheese Cake - Traditional 245
Pineapple Upside Down Cake 226
Quick Dump Cake 225
Spiced Sweet Potato Cake 227

CHICKEN

Aunt Era's Dumplings 203
Cajun French Chicken 101
Chicken and Asparagus 92
Chicken and Dressing - Light Recipe 250
Chicken and Dressing - Traditional Recipe 251
Chicken and Pasta 95
Chicken and Rice 96
Chicken and Snow Pea Salad 55
Chicken and Sun-Dried Tomato Sauce 99
Chicken and Yellow Rice 98
Chicken Asparagus Fettuccini 93
Chicken Divan 102
Chicken Paprika 111
Chicken Sauce Piquant 114
Chicken Spaghetti 116
Chicken Stew 117
Chicken Stir-Fry and Brown Rice 97
Chilled Chicken and Pasta Salad 56
Country Baked Chicken 100
Flakey Chicken Pie 112
Gravy for Chicken or Beef 31
Hawaiian Chicken Kabobs 103
Honey Glazed Chicken 105
Hot Chicken Salad 109
Lemonade Chicken 121
Lite King Ranch Chicken 108
Louisiana Chicken Jambalaya 106
Mexican Chicken Stew 118
New Orleans Style Chicken 110
Old Fashioned Chicken Salad 57
Ole South Coating Mix 30
Oven Fried Chicken 104
Potluck Chicken 113
Quick Chicken and Dumplings 94
Seafood Gumbo 46
Seafood Gumbo - Light Recipe 260

CHICKEN (Continued)

Sesame Chicken Kabobs 107
Smothered Chicken 115
Sportsman's Sauce 33
Springtime Asparagus Salad 53
Sweet and Sour Chicken 119
Sweet and Sour Marinade 31
Working Mother's Chicken 120

COOKIES

Low Fat Easy Bake Cookies 233

DESSERTS

Banana Pudding 238
Cherry Cobbler with Crumb Topping 229
Cherry Gelatin Delight 234
Elegant Ambrosia Compote 52
Flower Pot Dessert 233
Light Chocolate Brownies 231
Old Fashioned Lemon Squares 232
Orange Charlotte 235
Peach Cobbler 230
Quick and Easy Peach Cobbler 229
Quick Banana Pudding 239
Rice Pudding 240
Snow White Ice Cream - Light Recipe 246
Snow White Ice Cream - Traditional Recipe 246
Southern Blackberry Cobbler 228
Strawberry Dream 236

DIPS & DRESSINGS

Artichoke Dip 12
Light Crab Dip 13
Mama B's Thousand Island Dressing 29
Ole South Coating Mix 30
Picante Dip 14
Spinach and Cheese Dip 13
Spinach Salad Dressing 29
Tex Mex Dip 14

FISH

Baked Fish Au Gratin 77
Baked Red Fish 81
Bouillabaisse (Fish Chowder) 41
Courtbouillon 71
Courtbouillon (Koo-Bee-Yon) 72
Flounder Au Gratin 79
Grilled Fish Poboys 78
Ole South Coating Mix 30

FISH (Continued)
Oven Fried Catfish 70
Sportsman's Sauce 33
Stuffed Flounder 79
Stuffed Red Snapper 82
Tuna Casserole 91

GAME
Hunter's Venison Roast 153
Quail on Brown Rice 152
Tex Mex Venison Stew 154

PIE & PASTRIES
Deep Dish Strawberry Pie 237
Lemon Meringue Pie - Light Recipe 247
Lemon Meringue Pie - Traditional Recipe 248
Pecan Pie - Light Recipe 249
Pecan Pie - Traditional Recipe 249

PORK
Breakfast Biscuits 196
Hearty Potato Soup 44
Pork Chops and Vegetables 149
Seafood Gumbo 46
Smoked Ham and Cabbage 147
Southern Praline Ham 148
Stuffed Roast Pork Tenderloin 150
Sweet and Sour Marinade 31
Sweet and Sour Pork 151
Turnip Greens With Turnips 187

SALADS
Calico Mold 54
Cherry Gelatin Delight 234
Chicken and Snow Pea Salad 55
Chilled Chicken and Pasta Salad 56
Corn and Cucumbers 58
Easy German Potato Salad 64
Elegant Ambrosia Compote 52
English Pea Salad 62
Fresh Corn Salad 59
Fruit Salad 60
Hot Chicken Salad 109
Jack's Polka Dot Salad 57
Lime Jello Salad 60
Low Calorie Mandarin Orange Salad 63
Mexican Salad 61
Old Fashioned Chicken Salad 57
Red Potato Salad 65

SALADS (Continued)
Sea Shell Salad 66
Seven Layer Vegetable Salad 68
Springtime Asparagus Salad 53
Three Bean Salad 55
Turkey Delight 67

SAUCES
Bar-B-Q Sauce 26
Cheese Sauce 27
Cranberry Wine Sauce 28
Easy Salsa 27
Fat Free Hollandaise Sauce 28
Fat Free Roux 32
Gravy for Chicken or Beef 31
Medium White Sauce 34
Ole South Coating Mix 30
Southern Bar-B-Q Sauce 26
Sportsman's Sauce 33
Sweet and Sour Marinade 31
Thick White Sauce 36
Thin White Sauce 35

SEAFOOD
Cheesy Shrimp Noodle Bake 90
Crab Au Gratin 73
Crawfish Etouffee 74
Crawfish Pie 75
Crawfish Stew 76
Light Crab Dip 13
New Orleans Style Chicken 110
Ole South Coating Mix 30
Oven Fried Oysters 80
Oyster Bisque 39
Plantation Shrimp with Rice 83
Quick Seafood Gumbo 47
Sea Shell Salad 66
Seafood Casserole - Light Recipe 258
Seafood Casserole - Traditional Recipe 259
Seafood Gumbo - Light Recipe 260
Seafood Gumbo - Traditional Recipe 261
Seafood Lasagna 84
Shrimp and Angel Hair Pasta 85
Shrimp and Okra Creole 89
Shrimp Cocktail for a Crowd 20
Shrimp Corn Soup 50
Shrimp Creole 87
Shrimp Stuffed Bell Pepper 86
Shrimp with Eggplant Casserole 88

SOUP

A & W Bean Soup Mix 38
Bouillabaisse (Fish Chowder) 41
Cajun Gazpacho 42
Chicken Stew 117
Courtbouillon 71
Courtbouillon (Koo-Bee-Yon) 72
Crawfish Stew 76
French Onion Soup 48
Fresh Mushroom Soup 46
Hearty Potato Soup 44
Homestyle Chili 129
Instant Potato Soup 43
Jack's Bean Soup 38
Low Fat Vichyssoise 43
Mexican Chicken Stew 118
Oyster Bisque 39
Quick Seafood Gumbo 47
Seafood Gumbo - Light Recipe 260
Seafood Gumbo - Traditional Recipe 261
Shrimp Corn Soup 50
Split Pea Soup 49
Tex Mex Venison Stew 154
Turnip Soup 45
Vegetable Cheddar Chowder 40
Vegetable Soup 51

TURKEY

Baked Turkey Breast 121
Jack's Bean Soup 38
Left Over Turkey and Broccoli Casserole 122
Meat Pies 17
Quick Turkey Rollups 125
Sportsman's Sauce 33
Sweet and Sour Marinade 31
Turkey and Rice 123
Turkey Delight 67
Turkey Rollups 124

VEGETABLES & STARCHES

Baked Vidalia Onion 177
Braised Celery in Consomme 169
Broccoli Cheese Bars 10
Broccoli Cheese Casserole 163
Broccoli Cheese Roll-Ups 164
Broccoli Souffle 165
Broccoli-Cheese Potatoes 181
Broiled Fresh Asparagus 158
Cheese Grits 175

VEGETABLES & STARCHES (Continued)

Cheesy Sweet Onions 177
Corn Casserole - Light Recipe 252
Corn Casserole - Traditional Recipe 253
Corn Casserole with Tomatoes 171
Creamed New Potatoes 182
Creamy Cauliflower 168
Creamy Rich Noodles 176
Creole Eggplant 172
Dilled Yellow Squash 186
Fresh Snap Beans and Herbs 161
Garden Pilaf 174
Green Beans Dijon 158
Kahlua Carrots 167
Light Green Beans with Sour Cream 159
Mushroom Rice 176
Old Fashioned Baked Beans 162
Old Fashioned Whipped Potatoes 182
Oven Fries 179
Pleated Baked Potatoes 179
Quick Zucchini and Red Sauce 194
Red Beans and Rice 155
Scalloped Corn 170
Southern Garden Medley 173
Spicy Field Peas 178
Spinach Casserole 184
Squash Casserole 185
Summer's Delight 192
Sunday Green Beans 160
Sunshine Carrots 166
Sweet and Sour Vegetables 193
Sweet Potato Surprise 183
Turnip Greens With Turnips 187
Twice Baked Potatoes 180
Vegetable Bundles 188
Vegetable Lasagne 156
Vegetable Picante 191
Vegetable Vermicelli 190
Vegetables for a Crowd 189

Avis and Ward Nutrition Associates, Inc.
200 Professional Drive • West Monroe, La. 71291 • (318) 323-7949

_____ copies of **Gone With The Fat** $17.95 each $_____

_____ copies of **Southern But Lite** $17.95 each $_____

_____ copies of **Just For Kids** $12.95 each $_____

_____ aprons for **Just For Kids** $ 3.95 each $_____
(A cute Yellow/Gator child's apron–matches cookbook)
Louisiana residents add 4% sales tax. $_____

Shipping & Handling cookbooks $ 3.00 each $_____

Shipping & Handling aprons $ 1.50 each $_____

TOTAL ENCLOSED $_____
Make check payable to **Avis and Ward Nutrition Associates**

Please charge my: Visa _____ Mastercard _____

Card Number _____ Expiration Date _____

Send To:

Name: _____

Address: _____ Apt. _____

City: _____ State _____ Zip _____

- -

Avis and Ward Nutrition Associates, Inc.
200 Professional Drive • West Monroe, La. 71291 • (318) 323-7949

_____ copies of **Gone With The Fat** $17.95 each $_____

_____ copies of **Southern But Lite** $17.95 each $_____

_____ copies of **Just For Kids** $12.95 each $_____

_____ aprons for **Just For Kids** $ 3.95 each $_____
(A cute Yellow/Gator child's apron–matches cookbook)
Louisiana residents add 4% sales tax. $_____

Shipping & Handling cookbooks $ 3.00 each $_____

Shipping & Handling aprons $ 1.50 each $_____

TOTAL ENCLOSED $_____
Make check payable to **Avis and Ward Nutrition Associates**

Please charge my: Visa _____ Mastercard _____

Card Number _____ Expiration Date _____

Send To:

Name: _____

Address: _____ Apt. _____

City: _____ State _____ Zip _____